Sports Nutrition: More Than Just Calories – Triggers for Adaptation

Nestlé Nutrition Institute Workshop Series

Vol. 69

Sports Nutrition: More Than Just Calories – Triggers for Adaptation

Editors

Ronald J. Maughan Loughborough, UK
Louise M. Burke Bruce, Australia

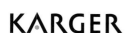

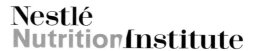

Nestec Ltd., 55 Avenue Nestlé, CH–1800 Vevey (Switzerland)
S. Karger AG, P.O. Box, CH–4009 Basel (Switzerland) www.karger.com

Library of Congress Cataloging-in-Publication Data

Sports nutrition : more than just calories - triggers for adaptation / volume editors, Ronald J. Maughan, Louise M. Burke.
    p. ; cm. -- (Nestlé Nutrition Institute workshop series, ISSN 1664-2147 ; v. 69)
  Includes bibliographical references and index.
  ISBN 978-3-8055-9697-8 (hard cover : alk. paper) -- ISBN 978-3-8055-9698-5 (e-ISBN)
  I. Maughan, Ron J., 1951- II. Burke, Louise, 1959- III. Series: Nestlé Nutrition Institute workshop series ; v. 69.
  [DNLM: 1. Nutritional Physiological Phenomena. 2. Sports--physiology. 3. Sports Medicine--methods. QT 260]
  LC classification not assigned
  617.1'027--dc23

                                                2011031957

Printed on acid-free and non-aging paper
ISBN 978–3–8055–9697–8
e-ISBN 978–3–8055–9698–5
ISSN 1664–2147
e-ISSN 1664–2155

Contents

Water

Concluding Comments

For more information on related publications, please consult the NNI website:
www.nestlenutrition–institute.org

Preface

Diet significantly affects athletic performance, and serious athletes recognize that adoption of a dietary strategy that meets their nutrition goals will maximize the possibility of competitive success. These goals, however, will vary between sports, at different times of the training and competition program, and between individuals.

The practice of sports nutrition has evolved over the years and has become increasingly complex. At one time, the focus was on achieving a high protein intake, especially a high intake of animal protein. This idea is intuitively attractive as it is easy to believe that a high intake of protein will support the building and repair of muscle proteins. In the latter part of the last century, the focus shifted. It was recognized that an adequate intake of protein is essential for all athletes, but the role of carbohydrate, especially muscle glycogen, and water became the focus of sports nutrition strategies. This reflected the recognition of the importance of carbohydrate availability and hydration status for performance in endurance performance in the laboratory. Ensuring a high dietary carbohydrate intake in training was encouraged for all athletes to allow consistent intensive training without the risk of chronic fatigue, illness and injury.

There is now a growing recognition that the primary role of sports nutrition may be to promote the adaptations taking place in muscle and other tissues in response to the training stimulus. There seems little point in training hard without taking advantages of the opportunities that nutrition support can offer. There is emerging evidence that the ingestion of relatively small amounts of protein, and more particularly of the essential amino acids present in proteins, before, during or soon after training can stimulate muscle protein synthesis, and that these effects may accumulate to amplify adaptations to training. Not all athletes want an increase in muscle mass, but remodeling of the muscle protein composition is as important for the endurance athlete as it is for the strength and power athlete. For athletes in sports with a high technical component, sound nutritional strategies may allow gains in strength and endurance with a smaller training stimulus, allowing more time to be devoted to the refinement of skills and technique.

There is also much interest in the implications of manipulation of the fat and carbohydrate content of the diet. It is well established that an adequate availability of endogenous carbohydrate stores is essential for performance, but it is also clear that nutrition strategies that spare carbohydrate use by increasing the oxidation of fat can enhance performance in events where carbohydrate is limiting. Various nutritional strategies that promote the capacity of the muscle to oxidize fat have been identified. Whether these can be adopted by athletes to enhance performance is less clear at the present time.

The aim of this workshop was to explore the effects of nutritional manipulations on the metabolic responses to acute and chronic exercise and to further identify the possible role of these dietary interventions in promoting adaptive changes in muscle, adipose tissues and other potential sites of limitation to exercise performance.

Ronald J. Maughan
Louise M. Burke

Foreword

Nutrition is central to a healthy active lifestyle. In fact, research has shown that physical activity, at the correct intensity and duration, not only improves the quality of life, it decreases the incidence of disease, chronic health conditions and obesity. For athletes, from elite active competitors to those who enjoy pushing themselves physically, diet has an important role to play in contributing to sporting success and activity goal achievements.

Life in the world of sport revolves around training and competition. To be able to healthfully sustain training, as well as strive for performance improvements, be it skill, power, strength, speed or endurance, recovery between training sessions is essential. Informed dietary choices help ensure fuel needs are met to promote adaptations to training, to facilitate a quick recovery to enable training to be continued and intensified, and to ensure good health. This workshop has explored the role of sports nutrition beyond mere calories to fuel training and competition, to its effect on triggering adaptive changes within the body.

The workshop, held in Kona, Hawaii, USA, in October 2010, brought together an exceptional group of scientific experts, all specialists in different areas of sports nutrition from around the world who contributed enormously to the lively and intense discussions. We are extremely grateful for their tenacity and energetic participation before, during and afterwards in helping make this workshop such a success.

Our special thanks go to the excellent chairpersons, Prof. Louise Burke from Australia and Prof. Ronald Maughan from the UK, highly respected experts in the field of sports nutrition and the practical application of dietary strategies for elite athletes, for putting together and facilitating this outstanding scientific program.

This publication includes all the presented scientific papers covering the three macronutrients: carbohydrate, fat and protein, plus an additional chapter on water, together with their accompanying discussions. For the first time, the discussion section of the Nestlé Nutrition Institute Workshop Series has changed its format. From now on, the discussion is compiled by an invited expert in the field. The concluding chapter summarizes the ways in which the technical scientific content from the workshop can be implemented as practical nutritional recommendations for athletes.

Quality of calories matter, and this 'quality' consideration is a particularly casing point for all athletes, whatever their level and whatever their goal, as revealed by the knowledge embedded within this book. Through the cooperation of the chairpersons with the Nestlé Nutrition Institute, an independent non-profit organization that fosters *science for better nutrition*, the proceedings of this Nestlé Nutrition Institute's Performance Nutrition Workshop will hopefully provide a useful contribution to the evolving science in the area of sports nutrition.

Prof. Ferdinand Haschke, MD, PhD
Chairman
Nestlé Nutrition Institute
Vevey, Switzerland

Dr. Samantha Stear, PhD
Global Science Lead
Nestlé Performance Nutrition
Florham Park, NJ, USA

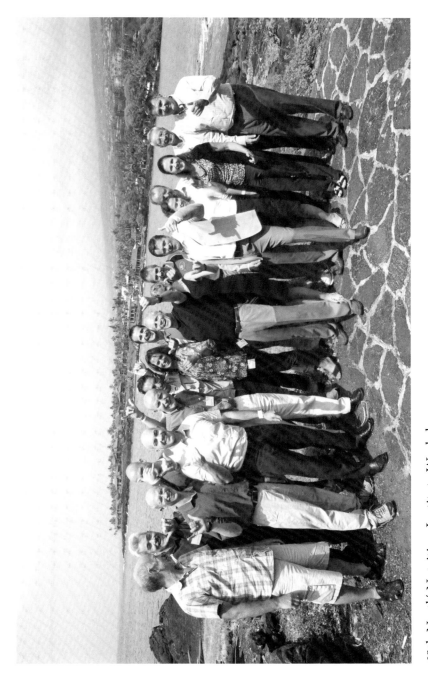

69th Nestlé Nutrition Institute Workshop
Kailua-Kona, Hawaii, October 7–9, 2010

Contributors

Chairpersons & Speakers

Dr. Keith Baar
1 Shields Ave
181 Briggs Hall
Davis, CA 95616
USA
E-Mail: kbaar@ucdavis.edu

Prof. Louise Burke
Sports Nutrition
Australian Institute of Sport
Leverrier Crescent
Bruce, ACT 2616
Australia
E-Mail: Louise.Burke@ausport.gov.au

Prof. John Hawley
RMIT University
School of Medical Sciences
Plenty Road
Bundoora, VIC 3083
Australia
E-Mail: john.hawley@rmit.edu.au

Prof. Asker Jeukendrup
School of Sport and Exercise Science
University of Birmingham
Edgbaston, Birmingham BT15 2 TT
UK
E-Mail: a.e.jeukendrup@bham.ac.uk

Prof. Florian Lang
Department of Physiology
Gmelinstr. 5
DE–72076 Tübingen
Germany
E-Mail: florian.lang@uni-tuebingen.de

Prof. Ronald Maughan
School of Sport, Exercise
and Health Sciences
Loughborough University
Loughborough LE11 3TU
UK
E-Mail: r.j.maughan@lboro.ac.uk

Prof. Stuart Phillips
McMaster University
Department of Kinesiology
1280 Main St West
Hamilton, ON L8S 4 K1
Canada
E-Mail: phillis@mcmaster.ca

Prof. Lawrence Spriet
Department of Human Health
& Nutritional Sciences
University of Guelph
Guelph, ON
Canada
E-Mail: lspriet@uoguelph.ca

Dr. Samantha Stear
Global Science Lead – Performance
Nutrition
Nestlé Nutrition R&D Centers, Inc
12 Vreeland Road, 2nd Floor,
Florham Park, NJ 07932
USA
E-Mail: samantha.stear@rd.nestle.com

Prof. Luc van Loon
Maastricht University Medical Centre+
PO Box 616
6200 MD Maastricht
The Netherlands
E-Mail: L.vanLoon@HB.Unimaas.nl

Invited Discussants

Prof. Martin Gibala/Canada
Prof. Hans Hoppeler/Switzerland
Prof. John McLaughlin/UK
Dr. Scott Montain/USA
Prof. Michael Zemel/USA

Nestlé Participants

Prof. Ferdinand Haschke/Switzerland
Ms. Laura Taylor/Switzerland
Ms. Patricia Griffin/USA

Maughan RJ, Burke LM (eds): Sports Nutrition: More Than Just Calories – Triggers for Adaptation.
Nestlé Nutr Inst Workshop Ser, vol 69, pp 1–17,
Nestec Ltd., Vevey/S. Karger AG., Basel, © 2011

Carbohydrate Ingestion during Exercise: Effects on Performance, Training Adaptations and Trainability of the Gut

Asker E. Jeukendrup[a] · John McLaughlin[b]

[a]School of Sport and Exercise Sciences, University of Birmingham, Birmingham, [b]School of
Translational Medicine, Faculty of Medical and Human Sciences, University of Manchester,
Manchester, UK

Abstract

Carbohydrate feeding has been shown to enhance endurance performance. During exercise of 2 h or more, the delivery of carbohydrates to the muscle is the crucial step and appears to be limited by intestinal absorption. It is therefore important to identify ways to overcome this limitation and study the positive and negative effects of chronic carbohydrate supplementation. There is evidence that intestinal absorption can, at least partly, be overcome by making use of multiple transportable carbohydrates. Ingestion of these carbohydrates may result in higher intestinal absorption rates and has been shown to lead to higher rates of exogenous carbohydrate oxidation which can result in better endurance performance. It also seems possible to increase the absorptive capacity of the intestine by adapting to a high-carbohydrate diet. Carbohydrate supplementation during exercise has been suggested to reduce training adaptations, but at present there is little or no evidence to support this. Despite the fact that it has long been known that carbohydrate supplementation can enhance endurance performance, there are still many unanswered questions. However, there is potential to develop strategies that enhance the delivery of carbohydrates and thereby improve endurance performance.

Introduction

The importance of carbohydrate as a fuel for exercise has been recognized since the early 1920s [1]. In particular, the availability of muscle glycogen has been linked to endurance exercise capacity [2, 3]. Ground breaking studies in the 1960s investigated the role of high muscle glycogen stores at the onset of exercise (carbo-loading) on exercise performance [2, 4–5], and in the 1980s the interest shifted towards the potential role of carbohydrate ingested just before and during exercise. Although the exact mechanisms are still not entirely elucidated, it is clear that carbohydrate ingestion during exercise can increase exercise capacity and improve exercise performance [for review, see 6–8]. Since the 1980s, studies have used a variety of exercise models to investigate the effects on performance of different feeding regimens, different types of carbohydrate and different amounts of carbohydrate. These studies have revealed the limiting steps for carbohydrate delivery to the working muscle, and this has resulted in new methods to increase this delivery. This review will focus on these recent studies as well as the mechanisms that limit exogenous carbohydrate oxidation during exercise and will discuss practical methods to overcome these limitations in order to improve exercise performance.

Carbohydrate Absorption

Before ingested carbohydrate can be oxidized by the working muscle, it has to be emptied from the stomach, digested (hydrolyzed unless ingested as monosaccharide) and absorbed. It then has to pass through the liver and be taken up by the muscle. Studies have repeatedly shown that gastric emptying is not the main limiting factor to delivery of carbohydrate to the muscle but it is beyond the scope of this paper to discuss the possible limitations and the evidence for and against in any detail. For more information, the reader is directed to other reviews [8, 9]. The most plausible explanation for the limitation to the oxidation of exogenous carbohydrate is that intestinal carbohydrate absorption cannot provide substrate to the working muscle at a high enough rate. This is in contrast to textbook statements which often indicate that the capacity of the intestine to absorb carbohydrate is 'virtually unlimited'. For example, Ferraris et al. [10] state that '...capacity for glucose absorption is one or two orders of magnitude higher than daily glucose intakes', while Crane [11] concluded that 'the total daily capacity is 10,211 g of a mixture of glucose and fructose; an amount equivalent to over 22 pounds of sugar and more than 50,000 calories'. The latter would equate to an average absorption of 7.1 g/min. Perhaps more realistic estimates were obtained from studies that used a triple lumen intestinal perfusion technique. Duchman et al. [12], having measured glucose absorption from a 6% glucose-electrolyte solution, estimated whole-body intestinal absorption rates to be in the range of 1.2–1.7 g/min. The measurements were made over a very short (40 cm) section of the gut, and extrapolations to whole-body absorption rates can therefore be problematic, especially because various parts of the gut have different absorptive capacities.

Intestinal sugar transporters are responsible for transporting the monosaccharide carbohydrates glucose, fructose and galactose from the intestinal lumen into the blood. The sodium-dependent glucose transporter (SGLT1) is located in the apical brush border membrane, and is responsible for the transport of glucose and galactose across the luminal membrane. Glucose and galactose are transported along with Na^+ from the lumen into the cytosol. For fructose, there is another transporter protein (GLUT5) that transports the sugar from the lumen into the cytosol, and this process is independent of Na^+. Both these transporters are present in the apical membrane and were discovered and cloned in the 1980s [13–15]. In the basolateral membrane, another transporter (GLUT2) is responsible for transporting the three monosaccharides from the cytosol into the blood. It is generally thought that the transporters on the luminal side are rate limiting. Studies using triple lumen technique or in vitro preparations of the gut may give information about the maximum absorptive capacity of a small section of the intestine, but these findings may be difficult to translate to an in vivo situation [16], particularly in the context of exercise. Perhaps the most insightful information has come from studies that have used stable isotope tracers to measure exogenous carbohydrate oxidation during exercise. When a single monosaccharide carbohydrate is ingested, the oxidation rate of this carbohydrate does not normally exceed 1 g/min [9], perhaps because the SGLT1 transporter may become saturated [17]. When, in addition to glucose, a second monosaccharide that uses a different intestinal transport system, like fructose, was ingested, total carbohydrate oxidation rates were significantly higher. This provides indirect evidence that intestinal transport limits exogenous carbohydrate oxidation [17]. These findings will be discussed in more detail below.

Different Types of Carbohydrate

Isotopic (^{13}C or ^{14}C) labeling techniques have been used to study the efficacy of various ingested carbohydrates. This has provided insights about the time course of oxidation, and also made it possible to compare the oxidation of different carbohydrates. When carbohydrates are ingested from the onset of exercise and at regular intervals thereafter, oxidation of the ingested carbohydrate increases and typically reaches a plateau after 60–90 min. Originally, carbohydrates like glucose, fructose, galactose, sucrose, maltose and glucose polymers were studied. It was found that fructose was oxidized at slightly (4%) lower rates than glucose [18], and galactose oxidation rates were almost 40% lower [18–19]. More recently, it was found that high-molecular-weight glucose polymers were oxidized at similar rates to low-molecular-weight glucose polymer [20]. Therefore, it is unlikely that the rate of intraluminal enzymatic hydrolysis of polysaccharides is limiting. In addition, it was found that trehalose, a disaccharide formed by an α, α_1, 1-glucoside bond between two α-glucose units, and isomaltulose, an isomer of sucrose, were oxidized at lower rates than maltose and sucrose, respectively [21–22]. For a more complete overview of oxidation rates of different carbohydrates, the reader is referred to recent reviews [7, 23]. Perhaps the most striking finding was that in none of these studies did exogenous carbohydrate oxidation rates exceed 1 g/min (60 g/h) [for detailed review, see 6–8]. The significance of this observation is reflected in various guidelines including those of the American College of Sports Medicine in 2007 which state that athletes should ingest between 30 and 60 g of carbohydrate per hour during prolonged exercise [24].

We suggested that this apparent ceiling of 1 g/min was caused by a limitation in the absorptive capacity of the intestine [7]. As discussed above, glucose is absorbed through the sodium-dependent glucose transporter protein SGLT1. This transport protein in the brush border membrane has a high affinity for glucose and galactose but not for fructose [25]. We hypothesized that the limitation for exogenous carbohydrate oxidation was a saturation of the SGLT1 transporters in the brush border membrane of the intestine which may occur at high rates of glucose ingestion. The evolutionary norm is the ingestion of complex carbohydrate from which absorbable monosaccharide must be liberated by enzymatic hydrolysis: direct loading with ingested monosaccharide is not the condition for which the SGLT1 system evolved. Fructose absorption is not regulated by this mechanism because it is absorbed independently by a sodium-independent transporter GLUT5 [26]. The combined ingestion of these two sugars should therefore result in an increased total delivery of carbohydrates into the circulation and increased oxidation by the muscle. Already in 1995, Shi et al. [27] found evidence that ingestion of carbohydrates that use different intestinal transporters might increase total carbohydrate absorption. In a study by Jentjens et al. [17], evidence was obtained that exogenous carbohydrate absorption was also enhanced. Subjects in this study exercised for 3 h at a moderate intensity in a randomized crossover design, and ingested isoenergetic amounts of either glucose or a glucose:fructose mixture. The oxidation rates in the glucose trials peaked around 0.8 g/min, whereas the oxidation rates with glucose:fructose peaked at 1.26 g/min (see table 1). The studies were extended by studying different carbohydrate mixes such as glucose:sucrose:fructose, glucose:sucrose and maltodextrin:fructose and different ingestion rates [28–34].

These studies indicated that exogenous carbohydrate oxidation rates could be increased to as high as 1.75 g/min if glucose:fructose was ingested at an average rate of 2.4 g/min. However, from a practical point of view the most exciting finding was that a maltodextrin:fructose mix, which is not as sweet as the mixtures discussed above and therefore more palatable, was oxidized at very high rates [31]. Oxidation rates in this study reached 1.5 g/min at an ingestion rate of 1.8 g/min.

It is important to note that in order to benefit from a glucose:fructose mixture, it may be necessary to saturate glucose transporters in the intestine by ingesting sufficient quantities. When carbohydrate is ingested at rates of

Table 1. Summary of the advice for carbohydrate (CHO) intake during endurance events of different durations

Event	CHO required for optimal performance and minimizing negative energy balance	Recommended intake	CHO type	Glucose	Glucose + fructose
<30 min	no CHO required				
30–60 min	very small amounts	mouth rinse	most forms of CHO	●	●
1–2 h	small amounts	up to 30 g/h	most forms of CHO	●	●
2–3 h	moderate amounts	up to 60 g/h	CHO that are rapidly oxidized (glucose, maltodextrin)	○	●
>2.5 h	large amounts	up to 90 g/h	only multiple transportable CHO		●

The amounts recommended and the preferred type and blend of CHO depends on the duration of the event. When the absolute intensity is very low, these figures should be scaled down. A closed circle indicates 'optimal', an open circle indicates 'ok' to use.

0.8 g/min, saturation may not occur, and ingesting part of this carbohydrate as fructose may not result in higher exogenous carbohydrate oxidation rates [35]. However, although glucose was ingested at very low rates in one of the trials (0.54 plus 0.26 g/min of fructose), the oxidation rates for both carbohydrate drinks were the same! This indicates that in some cases glucose:fructose may be an advantage (at high ingestion rates), but there is no disadvantage when it is ingested at low rates.

It is important to note that recent work suggests that combinations of multiple transportable carbohydrates may also provide benefits in terms of gastric emptying and fluid delivery [34, 36, 37]. In one study, it was demonstrated that gastric emptying using the double sampling technique or a ^{13}C-acetate tracer technique was significantly faster with glucose:fructose than with an isoenergetic amount of glucose [37]. Several studies have demonstrated that deuterium appearance in the blood is faster when added to a glucose:fructose solution than to an isoenergetic glucose solution, suggesting faster fluid delivery [34, 36, 37]. It is possible that these effects of glucose:fructose combinations also contribute to the observed performance benefits that will be discussed below.

These studies clearly demonstrate that it is possible to achieve very high exogenous carbohydrate oxidation rates when multiple differentially transportable carbohydrates are ingested.

Exogenous Carbohydrate Availability to Support Endurance Performance

Although studies have consistently shown that carbohydrate can enhance endurance capacity and performance, there have been relatively few attempts to establish a dose-response relationship. The majority of the early studies provided 40–75 g carbohydrate/h and observed performance benefits. Ingesting carbohydrate at a rate >75 g/h did not appear to be any more effective at improving performance than ingesting carbohydrate at a rate of 40–75 g/h. It has been suggested that this is because ingestion of 40–75 g carbohydrate/h already results in optimum carbohydrate availability and ingesting carbohydrate at higher rates may not increase the bioavailability [38]. However, these early studies were not without limitations. In some of these studies, not only was the amount of carbohydrate different but also the composition of the carbohydrates and other ingredients in the drinks, making it difficult to study a true dose response. It is also possible that performance measurements used in some of these studies were not sensitive enough to pick up the small differences in performance that may exist when comparing two different carbohydrate solutions [39]. In a recent review, we concluded that the dose-response relationship was not immediately obvious from the early studies, and that relatively small amounts of carbohydrate can already result in enhanced performance [7]. We also suggested that it is likely that exogenous carbohydrate oxidation rates were positively related to exercise performance, i.e. the more exogenous carbohydrate is available to the working muscle the better the performance. In the last few years, evidence has accumulated in support of such a dose-response relationship and a link between exogenous carbohydrate oxidation and performance. Recently, a well-controlled dose-response study was performed in which 12 cyclists received carbohydrate (glucose) at a rate of 0, 15, 30 and 60 g/h [40] during 2 h of moderate-intensity exercise. This was then followed by a 20-km time trial to measure performance. In this study, a dose-response relationship was observed between carbohydrate intake and exogenous glucose oxidation and between carbohydrate intake and time trial performance.

In another study, subjects ingested 1.5 g/min of glucose:fructose or glucose during 5 h of moderate-intensity exercise, and it was observed that the subjects' ratings of perceived exertion tended to be lower with the mixture of glucose and fructose than with glucose alone, and cyclists were better able to maintain their cadence towards the end of 5-hour cycling [32]. Rowlands et al. [41] also reported reduced fatigue when ingesting a maltodextrin:fructose mix. It was also demonstrated that a glucose:fructose drink could improve exercise performance [42]. Cyclists exercised for 2 h on a cycle ergometer at 54% VO_{2max}. During the exercise, they ingested either a carbohydrate drink or placebo, and were then asked to perform a time trial that lasted approximately another 60 min. When the subjects ingested a glucose drink (at 1.8 g/min), they improved their power output by 9% (254 vs. 231 W). However, when they ingested glucose:fructose, there was another 8% improvement of the power output over and above the improvement by glucose ingestion (275 vs. 254 W). This is the first study to show that exogenous carbohydrate oxidation rates may be linked to performance and the first study to demonstrate a clear performance benefit with glucose:fructose compared with glucose [42]. These findings were reproduced by Triplett et al. [43] who found very similar performance improvements with glucose:fructose over glucose only. In a study by Stannard et al. [44], subjects were fed galactose, galactose:glucose (1:1) or glucose:fructose (4:1). Although it was not directly measured, based on a study in which galactose oxidation was determined [19], it would be expected that exogenous carbohydrate oxidation from the galactose drink would be lower (galactose is oxidized at significantly lower rates than glucose). Subjects exercise for 2 h at 65% VO_{2max} followed by a self-paced time trial. Galactose ingestion resulted in significantly lower power outputs than the two other drinks, and this would support a link between exogenous carbohydrate oxidation and performance [44].

A large-scale multicentre study by Smith et al. [45] also investigated the relationship between carbohydrate ingestion rate and cycling time trial performance to identify a range of carbohydrate ingestion rates that would enhance performance. In their study, 51 cyclists and triathletes across four research sites completed four exercise sessions consisting of a 2-hour constant load ride at a moderate to high intensity. Twelve different beverages (three at each site) were tested providing participants with 10, 20, 30, 40, 50, 60, 70, 80, 90, 100, 110, and 120 g carbohydrate/h during the constant load ride. A common placebo that was artificially sweetened, colored, and flavored and did not contain carbohydrate was tested at all four sites. The order of the beverage treatments was randomized at each site. Immediately following the constant load ride, participants completed a simulated 20-km time trial as quickly as possible. The ingestion of carbohydrate significantly improved performance and the authors concluded that the greatest performance enhancement was seen at an ingestion rate between 60–80 g carbohydrate/h.

These findings challenge the current American College of Sports Medicine guidelines [46] which suggest that a carbohydrate intake of 30–60 g/h is optimal. Recent evidence seems to indicate that a higher intake of 60–80 g/h is optimal, and that perhaps even higher intakes may be better when multiple transportable carbohydrates are ingested. Recommendations by the authors are summarized in table 1.

Gut Adaptation

Since the absorption of carbohydrate limits exogenous carbohydrate oxidation, and exogenous carbohydrate oxidation seems to be linked to exercise performance, an obvious question is whether it is possible to increase the absorptive capacity of the gut. Anecdotal evidence in athletes would suggest that the gut is trainable and that individuals who regularly consume carbohydrate or have a high daily carbohydrate intake have an increased capacity to empty carbohydrate from the stomach and absorb it. From animal studies it would appear that this is indeed the case. It has been demonstrated that the intestinal carbohydrate transporters can be upregulated by exposing an animal to a high-carbohydrate diet [26, 47]. The mechanisms for this effect are unclear, but interesting animal data indicate a role for the sweet taste family (T1R) of G-protein-coupled receptors and signal transduction molecules such as a-gustducin [48]. Consequently, artificial sweeteners may provide the same responses [49]. The enteroendocrine cell population is the most likely site of nutrient sensing, but data functionally coupling these sensors to similar physiological effects in humans are currently lacking.

To date, there is limited evidence in humans to support or refute this theory. A recent study by Cox et al. [50] investigated whether altering daily carbohydrate intake affects substrate oxidation and in particular exogenous carbohydrate oxidation. It was hypothesized that when exposed to a high-carbohydrate diet for a prolonged period of time (28 days), carbohydrate transporters in the intestine would be upregulated, and this would result in an increase in exogenous carbohydrate oxidation during exercise. In order to study this, the investigators recruited 16 subjects and divided them into a high carbohydrate and a low carbohydrate group. Both groups were fed a diet containing 5 g/kg carbohydrate per day, but the high carbohydrate group received supplements providing an additional 1.5 g/kg carbohydrate per day. Before and after the 28-day period, exogenous carbohydrate oxidation was measured during a 100-min steady-state trial around 70% VO_2 peak. During the exercise bout, the subjects received a 10% glucose solution at 20-min intervals providing almost 2 g of carbohydrate per minute. Exogenous carbohydrate oxidation rates were higher after the high carbohydrate diet, providing evidence that the gut is indeed adaptable and this can be used as a practical method to increase exogenous carbohydrate oxidation. We recently suggested that this may be highly relevant to the endurance athlete and may be a prerequisite for the first person to break the 2 h marathon barrier [51].

Training Adaptation with Low Exogenous Carbohydrate Availability

Carbohydrate supplementation during exercise may not have only positive effects. The positive effects may refer to the acute situation but chronic use might have negative effects. It has been suggested that carbohydrate ingestion during exercise may limit training adaptations. This idea stems from observations that muscle glycogen stores are related to expression of genes relevant to the adaptation to training. It is generally thought that training adaptations are the result of recurrent changes in gene expression, which occur with every bout of exercise, leading to a change in phenotype such as increases in fatty acid transport and oxidation. For example, a single bout of exercise increases muscle mRNA content of peroxisome proliferator-activated receptor-γ coactivator 1α, a transcriptional regulator of mitochondrial biogenesis.

Chronic glucose ingestion might negatively affect the expression of relevant genes. Glucose ingestion can attenuate the rise in AMP-activated kinase (AMPK) [52], and chronic suppression of AMPK in turn could reduce the increase in citrate synthase activity [53] and reduce muscle glycogen accumulation [54], two well-known training adaptations. Glucose ingestion will suppress lipolysis and reduce the concentration of fatty acids in the plasma, and this possibly attenuate some of the training-induced adaptations. It has been shown that glucose ingestion during exercise may suppress the expression of CPT-1 mRNA, mitochondrial uncoupling protein (UCP3-3) and FAT/CD36 [55]. However, in a carefully conducted study by Akerstrom et al. [56] in which a 10-week leg extension training program was followed by the subjects, glucose ingestion did not alter training adaptations related to substrate metabolism, mitochondrial enzyme activity, glycogen content or performance. Significant increases were observed in citrate synthase activity and β-hydroxyl acyl-CoA dehydrogenase activity after the 10-week training program, but there was no effect of carbohydrate supplementation on these changes. It appears that the effects of glucose ingestion during exercise are distinctly different from those induced by exercising with low glycogen. Performing 50% of all exercise training in a low glycogen condition has been demonstrated to produce marked improvements in markers of oxidative capacity [57–59] compared with training in a glycogen-loaded state all the time.

Practical Implications

When exercise lasts for up to 2 h, a carbohydrate intake up to about 60 g could be recommended. When the exercise lasts 2 h or more, slightly greater amounts of carbohydrate (90 g/h) would be recommended, and these carbohydrates should consist of a mix of multiple transportable carbohydrates, e.g. glucose:fructose or maltodextrin:fructose. The source or form of these carbohydrates may not matter as much as previously thought. It was recently demonstrated that carbohydrates in a beverage were oxidized at similar rates to carbohydrates from a gel (semi-solid) [60]. Also, it was demonstrated that carbohydrates from a bar that contained mostly monosaccharide (in the form of glucose:fructose) could result in exogenous carbohydrates oxidation that are similar to those seen with a beverage [61]. Exogenous carbohydrate oxidation rates were not different during cycling compared with running [62], and therefore the advice would not be different for these two types of exercise.

In summary, in order to obtain a carbohydrate intake of 90 g/h, athletes could 'mix and match' to fulfill their personal preferences and take into account their tolerance. Of course, these practices have to be tried and tested. Interindividual differences, the effects of gender, habitual diet and nutrient sensing mechanisms all need to be evaluated. Since the gut is so adaptable, it seems wise to have a high carbohydrate intake during training and regularly ingest carbohydrate during exercise. With these strategies, the gut may be trained to absorb and oxidize more carbohydrate, which in turn could result in less gastrointestinal distress and better performance.

References

1   Krogh A, Lindhard J: The relative value of fat and carbohydrate as sources of muscular energy. Biochem J 1920;14:290–363.
2   Bergström J, Hermansen L, Hultman E, Saltin B: Diet, muscle glycogen and physical performance. Acta Physiol Scand 1967;71:140–150.
3   Rodriguez NR, Di Marco NM, Langley S: American College of Sports Medicine position stand. Nutrition and athletic performance. Med Sci Sports Exerc 2009;41:709–731.
4   Hultman E: Physiological role of muscle glycogen in man, with special reference to exercise. Circ Res 1967;10:I-99–I-114.
5   Hultman E, Bergstrom J: Muscle glycogen synthesis in relation to diet studied in normal subjects. Acta Med Scand 1967;182:109–117.
6   Jeukendrup A, Tipton KD: Legal nutritional boosting for cycling. Curr Sports Med Rep 2009;8:186–191.
7   Jeukendrup A: Carbohydrate feeding during exercise. Eur J Sport Sci 2008;8:77–86.
8   Jeukendrup AE: Carbohydrate intake during exercise and performance. Nutrition 2004;20:669–677.
9   Jeukendrup AE, Jentjens R: Oxidation of carbohydrate feedings during prolonged exercise: current thoughts, guidelines and directions for future research. Sports Med 2000;29:407–424.
10 Ferraris RP, Yasharpour S, Lloyd KC, et al: Luminal glucose concentrations in the gut under normal conditions. Am J Physiol 1990;259:G822–G837.
11 Crane RK: The physiology of the intestinal absorption of sugars; in Jeanes A, Hodge J (eds): Physiological Effects of Food Carbohydrates. Washington, American Chemical Society, 1975.
12 Duchman SM, Ryan AJ, Schedl HP, et al: Upper limit for intestinal absorption of a dilute glucose solution in men at rest. Med Sci Sports Exerc 1997;29:482–488.
13 Hediger MA, Coady MJ, Ikeda TS, Wright EM: Expression cloning and cDNA sequencing of the Na^+/glucose co-transporter. Nature 1987;330:379–381.
14 Thorens B, Sarkar HK, Kaback HR, Lodish HF: Cloning and functional expression in bacteria of a novel glucose transporter present in liver, intestine, kidney, and beta-pancreatic islet cells. Cell 1988;55:281–290.
15 Burant CF, Takeda J, Brot-Laroche E, et al: Fructose transporter in human spermatozoa and small intestine is GLUT5. J Biol Chem 1992;267:14523–14526.
16 Gisolfi CV, Summers RW, Schedl HP, et al: Human intestinal water absorption: direct vs. indirect measurements. Am J Physiol 1990;258:G216–G222.

17 Jentjens RL, Moseley L, Waring RH, et al: Oxidation of combined ingestion of glucose and fructose during exercise. J Appl Physiol 2004;96:1277–1284.

18 Burelle Y, Lamoureux MC, Peronnet F, et al: Comparison of exogenous glucose, fructose and galactose oxidation during exercise using 13C-labelling. Br J Nutr 2006;96:56–61.

19 Leijssen DP, Saris WH, Jeukendrup AE, Wagenmakers AJ: Oxidation of exogenous [^{13}C]galactose and [^{13}C]glucose during exercise. J Appl Physiol 1995;79:720–725.

20 Rowlands DS, Wallis GA, Shaw C, et al: Glucose polymer molecular weight does not affect exogenous carbohydrate oxidation. Med Sci Sports Exerc 2005;37:1510–1516.

21 Venables MC, Brouns F, Jeukendrup AE: Oxidation of maltose and trehalose during prolonged moderate-intensity exercise. Med Sci Sports Exerc 2008;40:1653–1659.

22 Achten J, Jentjens RL, Brouns F, Jeukendrup AE: Exogenous oxidation of isomaltulose is lower than that of sucrose during exercise in men. J Nutr 2007;137:1143–1148.

23 Jeukendrup AE: Carbohydrate and exercise performance: the role of multiple transportable carbohydrates. Curr Opin Clin Nutr Metab Care 2010;13:452–457.

24 American College of Sports Medicine, Sawka MN, Burke LM, Eichner ER, et al: American College of Sports Medicine position stand. Exercise and Fluid Replacement. Med Sci Sports Exerc 2007;39:377–390.

25 Kellett GL: The facilitated component of intestinal glucose absorption. J Physiol 2001;531:585–595.

26 Ferraris RP, Diamond J: Regulation of intestinal sugar transport. Physiol Rev 1997;77:257–302.

27 Shi X, Summers RW, Schedl HP, et al: Effects of carbohydrate type and concentration and solution osmolality on water absorption. Med Sci Sports Exerc 1995;27:1607–1615.

28 Jentjens RL, Venables MC, Jeukendrup AE: Oxidation of exogenous glucose, sucrose, and maltose during prolonged cycling exercise. J Appl Physiol 2004;96:1285–1291.

29 Jentjens RL, Achten J, Jeukendrup AE: High oxidation rates from combined carbohydrates ingested during exercise. Med Sci Sports Exerc 2004;36:1551–1558.

30 Jentjens RL, Jeukendrup AE: High rates of exogenous carbohydrate oxidation from a mixture of glucose and fructose ingested during prolonged cycling exercise. Br J Nutr 2005;93:485–492.

31 Wallis GA, Rowlands DS, Shaw C, et al: Oxidation of combined ingestion of maltodextrins and fructose during exercise. Med Sci Sports Exerc 2005;37:426–432.

32 Jeukendrup AE, Moseley L, Mainwaring GI, et al: Exogenous carbohydrate oxidation during ultraendurance exercise. J Appl Physiol 2006;100:1134–1141.

33 Jentjens RL, Shaw C, Birtles T, et al: Oxidation of combined ingestion of glucose and sucrose during exercise. Metabolism 2005;54:610–618.

34 Jentjens RL, Underwood K, Achten J, et al: Exogenous carbohydrate oxidation rates are elevated after combined ingestion of glucose and fructose during exercise in the heat. J Appl Physiol 2006;100:807–816.

35 Hulston CJ, Wallis GA, Jeukendrup AE: Exogenous CHO oxidation with glucose plus fructose intake during exercise. Med Sci Sports Exerc 2009;41:357–363.

36 Currell K, Urch J, Cerri E, et al: Plasma deuterium oxide accumulation following ingestion of different carbohydrate beverages. Appl Physiol Nutr Metab 2008;33:1067–1072.

37 Jeukendrup AE, Moseley L: Multiple transportable carbohydrates enhance gastric emptying and fluid delivery. Scand J Med Sci Sports 2010;20:112–121.

38 Coggan AR, Swanson SC: Nutritional manipulations before and during endurance exercise: effects on performance. Med Sci Sports Exerc 1992;24:S331–S335.

39 Currell K, Jeukendrup AE: Validity, reliability and sensitivity of measures of sporting performance. Sports Med 2008;38:297–316.

40 Smith JW, Zachwieja JJ, Peronnet F, et al: Fuel selection and cycling endurance performance with ingestion of [13C]glucose: evidence for a carbohydrate dose response. J Appl Physiol 2010;108:1520–1529.

41 Rowlands DS, Thorburn MS, Thorp RM, et al: Effect of graded fructose coingestion with maltodextrin on exogenous 14C-fructose and 13C-glucose oxidation efficiency and high-intensity cycling performance. J Appl Physiol 2008;104:1709–1719.

42   Currell K, Jeukendrup AE: Superior endur-
     ance performance with ingestion of multiple
     transportable carbohydrates. Med Sci Sports
     Exerc 2008;40:275–281.
43   Triplett D, Doyle JA, Rupp JC, Benardot
     D: An isocaloric glucose-fructose bever-
     age's effect on simulated 100-km cycling
     performance compared with a glucose-only
     beverage. Int J Sport Nutr Exerc Metab
     2010;20:122–131.
44   Stannard SR, Hawke EJ, Schnell N: The effect
     of galactose supplementation on endur-
     ance cycling performance. Eur J Clin Nutr
     2009;63:209–214.
45   Smith JW, Zachwieja JJ, Horswill CA, et al:
     Evidence of a carbohydrate dose and pro-
     longed exercise performance relationship.
     Med Sci Sports Exerc 2010;42:84.
46   Joint Position Statement: nutrition and
     athletic performance. American College
     of Sports Medicine, American Dietetic
     Association, and Dietitians of Canada. Med
     Sci Sports Exerc 2000;32:2130–2145.
47   Ferraris RP: Dietary and developmental
     regulation of intestinal sugar transport.
     Biochem J 2001;360:265–276.
48   Dyer J, Daly K, Salmon KS, et al: Intestinal
     glucose sensing and regulation of intestinal
     glucose absorption. Biochem Soc Trans
     2007;35:1191–1194.
49   Moran AW, Al-Rammahi MA, Arora DK, et
     al: Expression of Na$^+$/glucose co-transporter
     1 (SGLT1) is enhanced by supplementation
     of the diet of weaning piglets with artificial
     sweeteners. Br J Nutr 2010;104:637–646.
50   Cox GR, Clark SA, Cox AJ, et al: Daily
     training with high carbohydrate availability
     increases exogenous carbohydrate oxidation
     during endurance cycling. J Appl Physiol
     2010;109:126–134.
51   Stellingwerff T, Jeukendrup AE, Perrey
     S, et al: Commentaries on viewpoint: the
     two-hour marathon: who and when? J Appl
     Physiol 2011;110:278–293.
52   Akerstrom TC, Birk JB, Klein DK, et al: Oral
     glucose ingestion attenuates exercise-induced
     activation of 5′-AMP-activated protein
     kinase in human skeletal muscle. Biochem
     Biophys Res Commun 2006;342:949–955.
53   Winder WW, Holmes BF, Rubink DS, et al:
     Activation of AMP-activated protein kinase
     increases mitochondrial enzymes in skeletal
     muscle. J Appl Physiol 2000;88:2219–2226.
54   Holmes BF, Kurth-Kraczek EJ, Winder WW:
     Chronic activation of 5′-AMP-activated
     protein kinase increases GLUT-4, hexoki-
     nase, and glycogen in muscle. J Appl Physiol
     1999;87:1990–1995.
55   Civitarese AE, Hesselink MK, Russell AP, et
     al: Glucose ingestion during exercise blunts
     exercise-induced gene expression of skeletal
     muscle fat oxidative genes. Am J Physiol
     Endocrinol Metab 2005;289:E1023–E1029.
56   Akerstrom TCA, Fischer CP, Plomgaard P,
     et al: Glucose ingestion during endurance
     training does not alter adaptation. J Appl
     Physiol 2009;106:1771–1779.
57   Hulston CJ, Venables MC, Mann CH, et al:
     Training with low muscle glycogen enhances
     fat metabolism in well-trained cyclists. Med
     Sci Sports Exerc 2010;42:2046–2055.
58   Yeo WK, Paton CD, Garnham AP, et al:
     Skeletal muscle adaptation and performance
     responses to once a day versus twice every
     second day endurance training regimens.
     J Appl Physiol 2008;105:1462–1470.
59   Hansen AK, Fischer CP, Plomgaard P, et al:
     Skeletal muscle adaptation: training twice
     every second day vs. training once daily.
     J Appl Physiol 2005;98:93–99.
60   Pfeiffer B, Stellingwerff T, Zaltas E,
     Jeukendrup AE: CHO oxidation from a CHO
     gel compared with a drink during exercise.
     Med Sci Sports Exerc 2010;42:2038–2045.
61   Pfeiffer B, Stellingwerff T, Zaltas E,
     Jeukendrup AE: Oxidation of solid versus
     liquid CHO sources during exercise. Med Sci
     Sports Exerc 2010;42:2030–2037.
62   Pfeiffer B, Stellingwerff T, Zaltas E, et al:
     Carbohydrate oxidation from a drink during
     running compared to cycling exercise. Med
     Sci Sports Exerc 2011;43:327–334.

Discussion

Dr. McLaughlin: In your presentation, carbohydrate ingestion is expressed in absolute amounts, in grams. Gastrointestinal effects, however, are linked more to concentrations. What volumes are being provided to achieve those intakes, and what is the osmolality of typical solutions?

Dr. Jeukendrup: The osmolality depends partly on the type of carbohydrate provided, but generally the osmolality of these solutions is high, especially when we give glucose and fructose mixes at rates of 1.5–1.8 g/min. We typically use solutions of 10–14% carbohydrate, which are a lot higher than the current recommendations, but similar to what athletes actually do in many endurance events.

Dr. McLaughlin: You comment that the mixture speeds up gastric emptying, but in healthy volunteers at rest, such concentrations will delay gastric emptying significantly. Is something different occurring in the exercising volunteers?

Dr. Jeukendrup: No, you are correct that higher carbohydrate concentrations reduce gastric emptying: These mixes will delay gastric emptying compared to a solution that is 6% carbohydrate. However, when we are talking about higher rates of carbohydrate intake and compare glucose alone with the multiple transportable carbohydrates, the latter will be emptied more quickly.

Dr. McLaughlin: Have you undertaken any measurements of the insulinemic response to these mixed carbohydrate preparations? It is inevitable that if you are increasing the amounts of carbohydrate absorbed in the portal system, insulin secretion is going to be enhanced.

Dr. Jeukendrup: Yes, although the exercise potently suppresses insulin secretion. Even though such prolonged exercise is undertaken at relatively low exercise intensities (typically ~60% VO_{2max}), circulating insulin levels are quite low.

Dr. Spriet: You discussed the Cox study in which well-trained athletes trained for a month with either a high or moderate carbohydrate intake, based on whether they consumed carbohydrates or water during each of their exercise sessions. You concluded that all of the adaptation to the higher carbohydrate intake, which led to an improved ability to oxidize exogenous carbohydrate during exercise, occurred at the level of the gut. However, is there any reason why you would not expect some adaptation to take place at the level of the muscle as well? For example, if training is undertaken for just 2 or 3 weeks, clear increases in GLUT4 expression in the sarcolemma can be demonstrated.

Dr. Jeukendrup: Of course, I can't exclude that possibility, but my interpretation is based principally on the fact that the limitation of total exogenous carbohydrate oxidation capacity is not situated at the muscle level, but in intestinal absorptive capacity.

Dr. Burke: Can I add that there was no change in total muscle GLUT4 concentrations associated with the training and dietary interventions in this study?

Dr. Spriet: But of course, total protein content doesn't necessarily predict transport. You would need to isolate sarcolemmal vesicles and undertake transport studies in these vesicles.

Dr. Hawley: Is the training status from which athletes start important in designing and interpreting these experiments?

Dr. Jeukendrup: I don't think that the training status matters that much. My key message is the gut is the limiting factor, because the absorption capacity is saturable. We have generally done this study with subjects who are trained enough to be able to exercise for 2 h, but we have also compared relatively untrained with extremely trained and found absolutely no differences.

Dr. van Loon: You measure total carbohydrate oxidation, but are there differences in the metabolic fate of glucose and fructose? What is happening in the liver in particular?

Dr. Jeukendrup: We don't have the actual measurements, but glucose goes through the liver and is simply transported to the muscle to utilize. Fructose is handled differently, being converted mostly to lactate in the liver. It is the lactate that is transported to the muscle for use. You can clearly see much higher plasma lactate levels in any trial where fructose is administered.

Dr. van Loon: Is the lactate being used exclusively by the active muscle or by other tissues?

Dr. Jeukendrup: I would think because of the rate of utilization, it has to be utilized in active muscle.

Dr. Zemel: You commented on several genes, such as UCP3 and others that were downregulated. What is the time course of these experiments?

Dr. Jeukendrup: Usually mRNA abundances are measured, and if I recall from 2 or 3 studies, the downregulation happens almost immediately, and is maintained for a longer period of time.

Dr. Maughan: To return to Dr. McLaughlin's point about concentrations rather than amounts of carbohydrate, I think it's important to recognize that if you give a more concentrated carbohydrate solution, the liquid volume that is emptied from the stomach is reduced, but you still deliver more carbohydrate in total. So carbohydrate delivery to the small intestine is increased, but fluid delivery is decreased. The outcome of achieving very good carbohydrate transport with such hypertonic solutions in the small intestine is to induce water transport in the opposite direction. The initial studies which showed net secretion of water into the small intestine were done with segmental intestinal perfusion. Recently, however, we have done several studies where volunteers drink 10% carbohydrate solutions, and we can actually demonstrate a measurable decrease in plasma volume for the first hour or so after their consumption. So if a subject drinks 500 ml of a high-carbohydrate drink, they will secrete water into their gut lumen and be systemically more dehydrated after the drink than before it.

Dr. Haschke: Doesn't reduced urinary excretion compensate for this?

Dr. Maughan: That will happen later, but in the short term – that is, within 10 or 15 min of ingestion – there is a clear decrease in blood volume. Therefore, I think there are some other processes happening in the gut, and if we consider the practical implications for performance, we need to consider whether dehydration and a reduced circulating plasma volume is a significant issue.

Dr. Jeukendrup: That situation is probably most relevant for solutions containing mainly one type of carbohydrate. If the ingested drink has the multiple transportable carbohydrate mix, you would definitely improve fluid delivery and reduce this type of problem. In our studies, we haven't seen changes in relevant measurements such as plasma osmolality or hematocrit.

Dr. Phillips: With respect to the observation of suppressed gene expression following ingestion of the carbohydrate, is it possible that if subjects are simply able to do more work, they will overcome these effects? This would make it irrelevant in terms of phenotypic adaptation.

Dr. Jeukendrup: This is possible, of course. But sometimes, the exercise that is undertaken is too short to really notice an effect of carbohydrate intake. Some of these studies have used a 1-hour period, where one wouldn't really expect that ingested carbohydrate would make the exercise much easier. It's after 2 or more hours of exercise that we observe those effects.

Dr. Lang: What happens to the non-absorbed glucose? Inhibition of the sodium chloride-glucose cotransport may produce diarrhea. Do these athletes get diarrhea?

Dr. Jeukendrup: I think eventually that the carbohydrate will be absorbed.

Dr. Hoppeler: Is there an evolutionary limit to absorption? Although other animals such as dogs and goats have similar absorption rates, there are some species which can change gut physiology dramatically – such as migratory birds and snakes. There's a possibility that this adaptability is not realized in humans.

Dr. Baar: By contrast, hibernating animals are creatures that aren't using their gut for a long period. Are there any data to show changes in gut transporter function with these animals? It would also be interesting to compare what happens in bears that are vegetarian versus bears that are meat eaters: is there greater dependence in one situation than another?

Dr. Jeukendrup: I don't know that literature very well. But the migratory bird is an extreme example of very rapid regulation – they increase their capacity to take up ingested fat very rapidly.

Dr. Montain: My question has to do more with how this area of research could be applied to enhance adaptation. We have known for quite a while now that exogenous carbohydrate delivered during exercise can produce more power. If an athlete could use strategies every day in training to produce more power, they should get stronger over time. Is there any other aspect of this that could be exploited from your observation?

Dr. Jeukendrup: There is not really enough evidence to draw a really firm conclusion on whether it does or doesn't do anything. It may not do anything except help to maintain the exercise intensity, and I think that should at some stage be beneficial. However, I can't be sure.

Dr. Hawley: One of the things about being an athlete is that you have to stay healthy before you can get fit. What is the evidence for chronic carbohydrate ingestion during exercise having effects on health and the immune system?

Dr. Jeukendrup: We and others have conducted studies which show that markers of the immune system are better maintained when subjects consume carbohydrate during exercise. So, that could be another reason to adopt this approach, but I am not sure how important those markers really are in the overall scheme of preventing illness.

Dr. Maughan: I know your remit was to focus upon carbohydrate, but as the aim is to maximize exogenous substrates, is it timely to look at other nutrient types? A key one that comes to mind is acetate since there seems to be no barrier (at least in dilute solutions) to gastric emptying and absorption. Also, having considered the metabolic fate of fructose, why not consume lactate itself and bypass the need for metabolism in the liver? The gut's carboxylate transporters will rapidly absorb ingested lactate.

Dr. Jeukendrup: The practical problem is how to deliver acetate and lactate in large quantities. Although, in theory, lactate should work really well, tolerance to intake of large amounts of lactate salts hasn't been great in our trials to date. One solution would be to use polylactate, but this has been shown to be difficult to digest and therefore not very useful. Medium-chain triglycerides behave somewhat like carbohydrate, are energy dense, and according to our tracer studies, are oxidized very rapidly. The problem, again, is that tolerance is limited to small amounts only. We have found that if we give more than 30 g of MCT over a period of 2–3 h, this precipitates GI distress. Yet the delivery of 30 g is not enough to make a significant difference to energy intake, metabolism or performance.

Dr. Baar: Have you studied any anaplerotic amino acids, such as leucine or glutamine?

Dr. Jeukendrup: We have done a bit of work in this area, but there are quite a few studies now that have used studies that use branched-chain amino acids or amino acids in combination with carbohydrate. This has been an area of great discussion in the last few years with studies from Mike Saunders' and John Ivy's groups reporting benefits over carbohydrate. Several other studies, however, which have generally been better designed and incorporated better controls have failed to find these effects.

Dr. Spriet: If we consider alternate fuels such as acetate and lactate, or medium-chain triglycerides, it is frequently forgotten that the amount of energy derived is about half of that from nutritional glucose or long fatty acids. Secondly, it's quite easy to load the system with high concentrations of these things at rest, but during exercise, the biochemical pathways are not set up for this, even with lactate. Biochemistry doesn't favor moving from lactate to pyruvate in muscle under almost all situations, so the tissue is not able to oxidize that much of it.

Dr. Gibala: There are no events on the Olympic program which require exercise time to fatigue. What in your opinion is the best measure of performance?

Dr. Jeukendrup: This really depends on the question that you are trying to answer. The best performance test is the competitive event itself, but then the problem is the lack of a control trial. There is a time and a place to study time to exhaustion, which is relatively easy to do. I think this protocol comes from studies undertaken in animals where there aren't any other options, but it really measures aspects of fatigue. In humans, time to exhaustion depends on the individual's decision of when they have had enough of the exercise task, and there is a huge day to day variation. One does not see such variation in time trials. There is another problem, however, in that we are reliant on the subject's pacing strategies, and differences may be hard to pick up. Overall, I think in situations where you are really looking for a performance answer, you should probably do some form of true performance test such as a time trial. But if you want some measurements to look at the mechanisms at the same time, you could ask participants to do a fixed work load for some period of time then follow with a time trial. This is the protocol we've used the most over the last few years: 1.5–2 h of steady state exercise, followed by a time trial of about 1 h. It seems to be quite sensitive to detect the effects of nutritional manipulations.

Dr. Burke: A comment about measuring performance also serves to criticize our own work as well as that of others. Even though we try to map what is happening to mechanisms and outcomes with such hybrid models of fixed intensity work load and time trials, I still don't think we are really measuring what is important to the performance of elite sport. In many cases, it is not just the total elapsed time of a performance that matters. Rather, it is whether an athlete can respond to challenges that happen during events, such as being able to suddenly increase the tempo in a marathon to sub 3 min/km pace, to surge up a hill, or to sprint to the finish line. If our protocols don't test the athlete's ability to superimpose a very high intensity burst of activity against the background of their general pacing, we probably haven't measured what is really important.

Dr. Jeukendrup: That's why I have always said you have to know what you are looking for when designing the study. If one wants to look at basic mechanisms or metabolic changes, subjects have got to do some kind of steady-state exercise. If we want to look at performance, we have to undertake a performance trial. Ideally, we should completely separate these two domains and try to answer one question at a time rather than trying to answer two or more questions in one overcomplex study.

Dr. Burke: But even if we put a time trial component into a protocol, maybe within that time trial we need to induce some other perturbations?

Dr. Jeukendrup: You could do so, but the next step from that is to ask why we don't study a real race or try to simulate a real race. That would be an even better performance measurement.

Dr. Hawley: I would like to revisit the issue of carbohydrate ingestion and muscle glycogen sparing. Most of us are aware of the original studies showing that there is no glycogen sparing during cycling, although there are some indications of sparing if you look at individual muscle fibers or if the intensity alternates between low and high workloads. We haven't really revisited that question in this context of high carbohydrate doses. My suspicion is that under these conditions if we look at single figures there probably is glycogen sparing. Can you comment on this?

Dr. Jeukendrup: In the studies where we fed carbohydrate at rates of 2.4 g/min, which is not a practically applicable situation in real life, we do observe muscle glycogen sparing. We have only seen that occurring, however, in this set of conditions. At intakes of 1.8 g/min, which is a little bit more realistic but still very high, glycogen sparing is not seen. You really have to push the system to see muscle glycogen sparing.

Dr. Hawley: Perhaps this might apply in an event such as the Tour de France where you are 'hiding' in the peloton for several hours at moderate workloads while ingesting mixed transportable carbohydrates at high rates. Then, as Dr. Burke pointed out, the high intensity bursts will be more effective.

Dr. Jeukendrup: Yes, it's very likely that muscle glycogen synthesis occurs in those recovery periods.

Dr. McLaughlin: A final comment on the human gastrointestinal system. We have about 8 m of small intestine and can lose most of it through surgical accidents or disease. Yet a residual couple of meters of small intestine can become completely adapted to fully absorb all the glucose that is required normally. So, it is clear that the capacity of the human gut for adaptation is absolutely enormous. However, the process is quite slow and can take years. One extra thing that is clear is that the presence of an intact colon is necessary for full adaptation after small bowel resection. We can therefore assume that some signals arise from the large intestine and feed back to the small intestine. Perhaps nutrient detection mechanisms operating within the small intestine are part of this system, and so other agents such as artificial sweeteners may also be able to stimulate these processes. There may also be other components, such as fiber, that the gut microflora acts upon which make an important contribution to adaptation. All these factors need to be taken into account in advancing this model.

Maughan RJ, Burke LM (eds): Sports Nutrition: More Than Just Calories – Triggers for Adaptation.
Nestlé Nutr Inst Workshop Ser, vol 69, pp 19–37,
Nestec Ltd., Vevey/S. Karger AG., Basel, © 2011

Altering Endogenous Carbohydrate Availability to Support Training Adaptations

Andrew Philp[a] · Louise M. Burke[b] · Keith Baar[a]

[a]University of California, Davis, Davis, CA, USA; [b]Sports Nutrition, Australian Institute of Sport,
Canberra, ACT, Australia

Abstract

Glycogen was first identified in muscle over a century and a half ago. Even though we have known of its existence and its role in metabolism for a long time, recognition of its ability to directly and indirectly modulate signaling and the adaptation to exercise is far more recent. Acute exercise induces a number of changes within the body (i.e. sympathetic nervous system activation and elevation of plasma free fatty acids) and muscle (increased AMP-activated protein kinase activity and fat metabolism) that may underlie the long-term adaptation to training. These changes are also affected by glycogen depletion. This review discusses the effect of exercise in a glycogen-depleted state on metabolism and signaling and how this affects the adaptation to exercise. Although 'training low' may increase cellular markers associated with training and enhance functions such as fat oxidation at sub-maximal exercise intensities, how this translates to performance is unclear. Further research is warranted to identify situations both in health and athletic performance where training with low glycogen levels may be beneficial. In the meantime, athletes and coaches need to weigh the pros and cons of training with low carbohydrate within a periodized training program.

Copyright © 2011 Nestec Ltd., Vevey/S. Karger AG, Basel

Introduction

In 1858 [1], Claude Bernard reported the successful isolation of carbohydrate from liver and muscle. This discovery began a century and half of research aimed at determining the function and clinical relevance of these cellular carbohydrate stores. The principal storage form of carbohydrate in mammals is glycogen, a polymer of D-glycosyl units joined by 1:4 or 1:6 bonds to produce a polysaccharide 'tree'.

The structure and metabolic regulation of glycogen has been the focus of researchers in many different fields [2]. Prior to the 1930s, glycogenolysis was thought to occur by simple hydrolysis of glycogen to glucose [2]. However, in 1936, Parnas and Ostern [3] demonstrated that it was more complex, requiring inorganic phosphate and resulting in the release of a hexose monophosphate 90% of the time and free glucose only 10% of the time. Carl and Gerty Cori identified the hexose monophosphate as glucose-1-phosphate, identified the enzyme that catalyzed this reaction as glycogen phosphorylase, and showed that the breakdown of glycogen was controlled by a series of reactions that required phosphate transfer [4]. For this work, which revolutionized our understanding of the physiological regulation of glycogen and introduced the first signaling cascade, the Coris, along with Prof. Bernardo Houssay, received the Nobel Prize in 1947.

Almost a century on from Bernard's landmark paper, Bergstrom and Hultman began to investigate the relationship between glycogen and exercise performance, and the mechanism of glycogen resynthesis following depletion [5]. These early studies demonstrated that the glycogen content of the working muscle is a major determinant of the capacity to sustain long-duration exercise [5]. Importantly, Hultman and Bergstrom [6] also demonstrated that alterations in diet and exercise could greatly vary the glycogen content in skeletal muscle, which then affected exercise sustainability. Finally, they observed that ingestion of a high-carbohydrate diet following exercise increased the recovery of muscle glycogen stores compared to a diet containing mainly fat and protein, providing direct evidence that dietary glucose was the precursor for muscle glycogen [7]. The increase in exercise performance with increasing glycogen has been replicated on numerous occasions [8] and has led to widespread changes in the nutrition of athletes.

Training with Low Glycogen: The Molecular Viewpoint

When glycogen availability decreases, whole body metabolism shifts dramatically. In humans, glycogen depletion results in reduced pyruvate oxidation, increased systemic release of amino acids from muscle proteolysis, and increased fat metabolism [9]. The decrease in glycogen content with exercise occurs concomitant with an increase in fatty acid oxidation, suggesting that lower glycogen is directly sensed by the body and leads to a shift in metabolism from carbohydrate to fatty acids. Furthermore, the transient decrease in muscle glycogen with exercise may be directly involved in the cellular adaptation to training by controlling signaling pathways within the active muscle [10].

Philp · Burke · Baar

To directly test the postulate that glycogen depletion is related to the muscular adaptation to training, Hansen et al. [11], hypothesized that training in a low glycogen state would provide greater muscle adaptation than the equivalent training in a normal or high glycogen state. In support of the hypothesis, a leg that started half of its sessions with low muscle glycogen concentrations over 10 weeks of training showed a greater increase in time to exhaustion and citrate synthase activity, and a trend towards higher 3-hydroxyacyl-CoA dehydrogenase activity (βHAD) than the subject's other leg that trained with high glycogen. The results of this study have since been extended to trained athletes [12, 13]. As would be expected, athletes who commenced high-intensity intervals with ~50% lower muscle glycogen showed significantly lower power outputs during each training bout than a cohort who exercised with higher glycogen content. However, 60-min time trial performance improved to the same degree following 3 weeks of training in both the cyclists who 'trained low' for half their sessions and cyclists who refueled between their training sessions. The major difference between the two training groups was in submaximal exercise, where following training, the low glycogen group used a significantly higher percentage of fatty acids and a significantly smaller amount of glycogen. Interestingly, tracer analysis indicated that the greater fat oxidation was the result of the increased oxidation of intramuscular triglycerides (IMTG), facilitated by increases in cluster of differentiation (CD36) protein and βHAD protein and activity. Together, these data indicate that regardless of training state, high-intensity exercise with low muscle glycogen improves the capacity for fatty acid oxidation to a greater degree than training with normal glycogen levels.

Manipulating glycogen stores creates a number of alterations that together are likely to underpin the improved adaptive response to training. These include changes in sympathetic nervous system activity, changes in the activity of proteins that contain a glycogen-binding domain, and alterations in fat and carbohydrate metabolism. Even though the exact molecular mechanism has yet to be determined, the existing data are sufficient to develop salient hypotheses as to how exercise in a low glycogen state drives improved fatty acid oxidation.

The key components of this paradigm (described below) are the peroxisome proliferator-activated receptor-γ coactivator (PGC)1α, the 5$'$AMP-activated protein kinase (AMPK), and the peroxisome proliferator-activated receptors (PPAR) α and δ (fig. 1). PGC1α is a coactivator of transcription factors involved in mitochondrial biogenesis, angiogenesis, and fat metabolism. AMPK is activated by metabolic stress, and acutely controls the rate of fat metabolism through its regulation of malonyl CoA levels and in the long-term alters transcription of genes involved in mitochondrial biogenesis and metabolism. The PPARs are fatty acid-activated transcription factors that, together with PGC1α, control the expression of enzymes of fatty acid metabolism. How the activity of these factors might be altered in a low glycogen state and work together to produce the enhanced training adaptation will be discussed below.

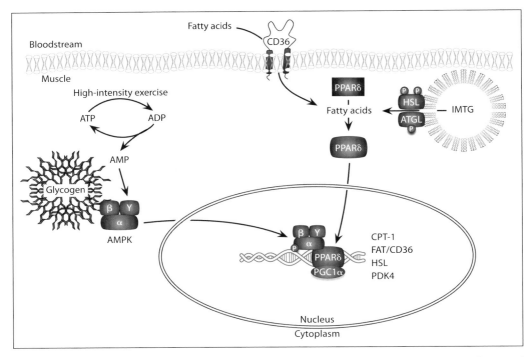

Fig. 1. Schematic diagram of the mechanism underlying the improvement in fatty acid oxidation following training in the low glycogen state. Low muscle glycogen increases catecholamine levels resulting in an increase in lipolysis and circulating fatty acids. Fatty acid uptake through FAT/CD36 combines with fatty acids from intramuscular stores (IMTG) to not only increase fat oxidation, but also bind to and activate the PPARs. Activated PPARs bind to the promoters of genes involved in fatty acid metabolism [carnitine palmitoyl transferase (CPT1), CD36, HSL, and pyruvate dehydrogenase kinase (PDK) 4]. Simultaneously, the lower glycogen levels result in higher AMPK activity following exercise. AMPK can bind to PPARδ and together with PGC1α transactivate PPAR target genes.

Exercise in a low glycogen state is perceived as a greater stress to the body resulting in elevations in circulating catecholamine (epinephrine and norepinephrine) levels, which can affect the adaptive response to training in two obvious ways. First, catecholamines can affect the adaptive response through the phosphorylation and activation of the cAMP response element-binding protein (CREB). Exercise can increase the activation state of CREB in both exercised muscle and muscles that were not recruited during the exercise [14] due to the elevated sympathetic nervous system activity. One of the targets of CREB is PGC1α. Akimoto et al. [15] demonstrated that the CREB site within the PGC1α promoter is required for the increase in PGC1α induced by exercise. Miura et al. [16] extended this work to show that blocking β-adrenergic receptors with ICI 118,551 prevented 69% of the exercise-induced increase in PGC1α.

Further, the induction of PGC1α following exercise was lower in mice lacking β-receptors than in wild-type mice [16]. Not only is PGC1α mRNA increased by catecholamines, catecholamines drive the expression of a splice variant of PGC1α made from a different promoter that may have a higher activity [17]. Together, these data suggest that catecholamines acting through β-adrenergic receptors may play a significant role in the increase in fatty acid oxidation following endurance training in the glycogen-depleted state. However, it should be noted that Mortensen et al. [18] showed that training in a low glycogen state did not alter the expression of the PGC1α family members in response to exercise, and Robinson et al. [19] did not see an increase in PGC1α expression or mitochondrial protein synthesis within the first 5 h after a 1-hour infusion of isoproterenol. However, it is not surprising that PGC1α mRNA is not changed after training (more likely after acute exercise) [18], and whether the primers used in these studies would identify the splice variant is unclear. Therefore, whether catecholamines can acutely regulate PGC1α in humans remains to be determined.

The second way catecholamines can increase the adaptive response to training is by altering fatty acid metabolism. Catecholamines alter fat metabolism by activating hormone-sensitive lipase (HSL) through protein kinase A (PKA). HSL is phosphorylated by PKA on three sites (Ser563, Ser659 and Ser660). Even though it is not clear how these sites regulate HSL activity, increased HSL activity drives lipolysis both in adipose tissue and skeletal muscle. The result is the liberation of free fatty acids from both fat and intramuscular depots. The increase in fatty acids delivered to the muscle during exercise results in an increase in the fatty acids oxidized for energy and an increase in the activity of the PPARs, transcription factors that are activated by binding to fatty acids. In muscle, PPARα and -δ, together with PGC1α, bind to the promoters of key enzymes of fat metabolism including carnitine palmytol transferase 1 (CPT1), CD36/fatty acid translocase (CD36/FAT), and HSL itself. We have recently found, in rats, that exercise in a glycogen-depleted state causes a greater increase in binding of PPARδ to the promoter of the CPT1 gene [unpubl. results], suggesting that PPARδ activity is increased and may underlie the improved phenotype following glycogen depletion training.

Mammalian AMPK is an αβγ heterotrimer with multiple genes encoding each of the subunits [20]. The regulation of the catalytic α-subunit is mediated by its phosphorylation, a glycogen-binding domain located on the β-subunit and the binding of AMP or ATP to the γ-subunit [20]. High-intensity endurance exercise increases α_2-AMPK activity up to 7-fold, whereas α_1-activity increases only ~50%. Beyond its greater activation by exercise, α_2-AMPK controls the metabolic adaptations associated with endurance exercise training. Mice that overexpress dominant negative α_2 do not undergo mitochondrial biogenesis in response to energy deprivation [21] and ablation of α_2-AMPK decreases basal and AICAR-stimulated expression of several metabolic genes in skeletal muscle and results in insulin resistance [22], suggesting that activation of α_2-AMPK promotes an endurance training phenotype. The tumor suppressor LKB1 appears to be the principal α_2-AMPK kinase in skeletal muscle since muscle-specific deletion of LKB1 reduces α_2-AMPK activity by ~95% [23]. We [unpubl. results] and others [24] have observed that both the basal and postexercise activity of α_2-AMPK is higher in the glycogen-depleted state. Furthermore, ingestion of sufficient glucose to spare glycogen depletion attenuates AMPK activation ~50% compared to a placebo trial [25], whereas a similar glucose ingestion protocol during cycling that did not result in glycogen sparing has no effect on α_2-AMPK activity [26]. This suggests that the amount of glycogen within the muscle directly modulates AMPK activity. In fact, McBride et al. [27] have shown that incubation of AMPK with isomaltose, which mimics the branch points of glycogen, inhibited the AMPK activity by 33%. Steinberg et al. [28] demonstrated that exercise in a glycogen-depleted state also led to nuclear translocation of α_2-AMPK and subsequent increases in GLUT4 mRNA expression. Nuclear translocation of α_2-AMPK has been suggested to be an important factor in the regulation of two important transcription factors: myocyte-enhancing factor 2 (MEF2) and nuclear respiratory factor 1 (NRF1). MEF2 and NRF1 play an important role in the control of a variety of genes for fiber type, carbohydrate metabolism, and mitochondrial biogenesis [29]. However, we demonstrated that the training-induced increase in GLUT4 protein was blunted when half of the training occurred in the low glycogen state [12], suggesting that AMPK alone does not underlie the low glycogen training effect.

Pharmacological studies by Narkar et al. [30] may provide an important clue as to how low-glycogen training can affect enzymes of fat metabolism. These authors showed that training rats on a treadmill while at the same time giving them GW1516, a drug that activates PPARδ, resulted in an increased capacity to use fat as a fuel. The GW compound alone had no effect on endurance or fat metabolism, whereas mice that were exposed to both the drug and training increased CPT-1, CD36/FAT and lipoprotein lipase, as well as their ability to run at ~50% of VO_{2max} more than those that just undertook training. Interestingly, when the GW compound was given together with AICAR, a drug that activates AMPK, the authors saw an increase in enzymes of fat metabolism. They also observed a direct interaction between α_2-AMPK and PPARδ and showed that the activity of AMPK and PPARδ could be increased a further 2.5-fold by PGC1α. Together, these data suggest that PPARδ interacts with AMPK and PGC-1α to increase the enzymes of fatty acid metabolism (fig. 1). When extrapolated to exercise in the glycogen-depleted state, these data suggest a possible mechanism for the improved adaptation: (1) exercise in the glycogen-depleted state increases circulating catecholamines; (2) catecholamines drive the transcriptional activation of PGC1α from its alternative promoter resulting in a more active form of PGC1α in muscle; (3) catecholamines also drive the breakdown of triglycerides to fatty acids resulting in higher plasma nonesterified fatty acids (NEFA); (4) increased NEFA and the breakdown of IMTGs results in greater uptake and oxidation of fatty acids; (5) the greater uptake and/or oxidation of fatty acids results in increased activation of PPARα and -δ; (6) high-intensity exercise in the glycogen-depleted state increases AMPK activity more than the equivalent exercise in a glycogen-replete state; (7) together, the highly active PGC1α, PPARs and AMPK bind to the promoters of genes involved in fatty acid metabolism and increase the expression of these genes; (8) when repeated, this results in an increased capacity to use fat as a fuel during exercise at 70% of VO_{2max}, sparing muscle glycogen, and potentially improving exercise capacity.

Training with Low Glycogen: The Athlete's Viewpoint

Clearly, the muscular adaptations achieved by training are an important part of improving athletic performance. However, changes in muscle physiology or cellular markers of metabolism are not, per se, a proxy for performance. Sports scientists are continually looking for strategies to enhance performance, and the elite athletes and coaches with whom they work stay up to date on cutting-edge research. Therefore, it is not surprising that news of the benefits of training with low glycogen [11] created a level of excitement in sports circles. Unfortunately, there is anecdotal evidence of misunderstandings by athletes, coaches and even sports scientists of the principles and practice of 'train low' techniques. Ill informed athletes are consuming carbohydrate-restricted diets for prolonged periods as a result of misunderstandings surrounding the train low strategy. However, the seminal train low study [11] neither implemented a carbohydrate-restricted diet nor exposed all exercise sessions to a low carbohydrate environment. Instead, their protocol and a series of follow-up studies have involved a 'two a day' training program supported by a carbohydrate-rich diet. The second training session in a day is undertaken a few hours following a first exercise bout whose goal is to deplete glycogen, with a short recovery period with negligible carbohydrate intake ensuring that there is minimal refueling during the recovery period. The second training session is then started with approximately 40% less muscle glycogen. However, in the recovery from the glycogen depleted session it is likely that there is super-compensation of muscle glycogen due to the subjects' high carbohydrate diet and the ~40 h of recovery before the next training session [31]. Other studies have used: (1) exercise after an overnight fast; (2) water only during prolonged training sessions; (3) carbohydrate-free periods in the hours after exercise, or (4) carbohydrate intakes below the fuel requirements of the training load [32]. These strategies differ in the duration of exposure to the low-carbohydrate environment as well as whether the glycogen is depleted locally (in the active muscle) or centrally (in the liver).

The clever design of the original study by Hansen et al. [11] involved previously untrained people who exercised one leg with a two a day training protocol every second day, while their contralateral leg undertook the same workouts spread over a daily training schedule. Ten weeks of training increased maximal power output equally in each leg, but the 'two a day' leg, which commenced half the training sessions in a low glycogen state, showed a greater enhancement of its capacity to work at ~90% of pretraining maximal power output. These findings have significant scientific merit and possible application for exercise programs targeting metabolic improvements and health outcomes. However, the relevance to athletic populations has been questioned on various grounds: (1) the large increase in metabolic capacity in previously untrained individuals compared with what would be expected from a well-trained population; (2) the relevance of the peripherally limited one-legged kicking exercise to sport, and (3) the use of a 'clamped' training program (each leg trained at the same absolute intensity in each session) in comparison to the principles of progressive overload and self-pacing that are incorporated into the training programs of athletes [32, 33].

Three further studies [12, 13, 34] have been undertaken utilizing the two a day model of training with low glycogen in athletic populations ranging from active to well trained. A variety of different parameters have been tested in these studies, including the type and volume of training, whether training was performed at a fixed intensity or according to a self-selected pace, and the protocol used to measure performance. It will take a large number of studies to cover all the potential areas of interest and application to sport. However, the general findings of this train low literature are consistent across all of the studies, namely that undertaking some exercise sessions with low muscle glycogen concentrations can enhance the metabolic adaptations associated with training, even in well-trained individuals. Muscle markers of aerobic metabolism are typically increased [12, 13, 34], and there is upregulation of fat utilization during steady state exercise [12, 13]. However, these benefits have not translated into a detectable performance improvement over conventional training with higher muscle glycogen concentrations [12, 13, 34]. Furthermore, the two studies in which the sessions completed with low muscle glycogen content were self-paced high-intensity interval workouts, self-selected power outputs were lower in the train low group than in the cohort undertaking a conventional training program [12, 13].

The possibility that train low protocols reduce the capacity to train at higher intensities/workloads requires attention. Most coaches prescribe training programs in which athletes are required to work at specific intensities/speeds/power outputs that are higher than their 'race pace' since success in most sports, including endurance and ultra-endurance events, is defined by high end speed (e.g. the sprint to the ball or finish line, the breakaway, the uphill climb, the surge). Intuitively, sacrificing the capacity to train at high intensities should be made with reluctance until there is evidence that this does not impair performance. Indeed, the performance benefits of training at moderate altitude, another strategy used to amplify training adaptations, were questioned when it was realized that high-speed training was compromised. As a result, altitude training is now performed differently: only during the base phase of training in which high-intensity training is less important, using 'live high, train low' (sleep at high altitude and train at lower altitudes) protocol, selecting a training location that provides access to a lower altitude venue where high-speed training sessions can be completed, or simply taking advantage of slight downhill sections that allow high-speed training at a lower metabolic cost. It should also be noted that unlike the endurance studies described above, the adaptations to resistance exercise are attenuated when the session is undertaken with low muscle glycogen content [35].

An important question from these studies is why the metabolic advantages in the muscle achieved by train low protocols have, in trained individuals at least, failed to transfer into performance benefits. Explanations for this apparent disconnect include the brevity of the study period, the length of the performance test (60 min or less) not benefiting from glycogen sparing, the possibility that performance is not reliant or quantitatively linked to the markers that have been measured [32] and the fact that as the intensity of exercise increases above 75–80% VO_{2max} during the performance test, there is a rise in epinephrine and a shift to carbohydrate metabolism regardless of the capacity to oxidize fat. Finally, there is the possibility that we may be unable to measure performance well enough in the lab to detect changes that would be significant in the world of sport [36]. It should also be noted that the performance trials used in the two studies most relevant to athletic training practices [12, 13] were undertaken following an overnight fast and without carbohydrate supplementation. This does not reflect the 'compete high' model originally proposed [11], or the current practices or sports nutrition guidelines for athletes [37].

Even though much of the discussion about low-glycogen training has focused on the benefits, it is important to consider the potential for side effects of this strategy as well. Apart from the potential loss of training at high power outputs/work rates, there is the possibility that upregulation of fat utilization during exercise is associated with downregulation of carbohydrate utilization. Indeed, in adapting to high-fat diets prior to carbohydrate loading for endurance and ultra-endurance events, the glycogen 'sparing' during exercise now appears to be the result of impaired glycogen use due to reduced pyruvate dehydrogenase activity, resulting in decreased carbohydrate entry into the TCA cycle [38]. This impairment in carbohydrate oxidation can impair the performance of sustained high-intensity activities during endurance events [39]. Finally, the effect of repeated training with low carbohydrate status on the risk of illness [40], injury [41] and overtraining [42] also needs to be considered.

Most elite athletes practice an intricate periodization of both diet and exercise loads within their training program that varies within a microcycle, e.g. over week(s) as well as over the year. Either by intent or happenstance, some training sessions are undertaken with low carbohydrate availability (overnight fasting, high volume training involving several sessions in the day, little carbohydrate intake during the workout), whereas others are undertaken with high carbohydrate status (more recovery time, post-meal, carbohydrate intake during the session) [32]. Therefore, in real-life, elite athletes already undertake a proportion of their training with low-glycogen content. It makes sense that sessions undertaken at lower intensity or at the beginning of a training cycle are most suited or perhaps least disadvantaged by train low strategies. Conversely, 'quality' sessions done at higher intensities or in the transition to peaking for competition are best undertaken with better fuel support. Athletes will, by accident or design, develop a nutrition strategy that suits their lifestyle and resources and maximizes their training and competition performances [32]. Finding this optimum balance is the art of coaching, and also the difficulty for sports scientists who need to conduct their studies with far more rigorous control than exists in real life. Furthermore, the milliseconds that differentiate the winners may result from things that cannot be measured in the lab.

Remaining Questions

The hypothesis that manipulating glycogen can optimize training adaptations is relatively new. As a result, there are a number of important questions that remain to be answered.

1 Is sympathetic nervous system activation required for the improvement in fatty acid oxidation following low-glycogen training? If catecholamines are important in regulating the expression of PGC1α from the alternative promoter, then high-intensity exercise will be a stronger stimulus for adaptation than the equivalent work completed at a lower intensity.

2 Are the PPARs, together with AMPK and PGC1α central to the improvement in fatty acid oxidation following low glycogen training? Is the response dependent on PPARα or -δ or do both isoforms function equivalently? These questions can be addressed using the PPAR-specific agonists: LY518674, fenofibrate, gemfibrozil, or troglitazone for PPARα and GW1516 for PPARδ. If, as expected, the PPARs play an important role in this adaptation, these agonists will have to be added to the banned agents list by WADA and other governing bodies for endurance competitions.

3 Is the increase in fatty acid uptake and oxidation key to increasing PPAR activity? If so, which endogenous ligands (fatty acids) best activate the PPARs? Are there nutritional strategies that can legally maximize the activation of the PPARs? For instance, green tea extract increases circulating fatty acid levels. Can green tea increase PPAR activation and the adaptive response to training?

4　What are the current training and nutrition practices of the world's best athletes, and how does this influence carbohydrate availability for each session in the microcycles and macrocycles of the periodized training program?

5　How can research protocols be designed to systematically study the range of possible permutations and combinations of train high and train low strategies within the periodized training programs of highly trained athletes, and thus identify ways to promote superior performance outcomes in specific sports?

Conclusions

The manipulation of pretraining muscle glycogen is a very easy way to optimize the capacity for fat oxidation following endurance exercise training. Low-glycogen training has the potential to not only provide a novel training technique for athletes, but it may also provide fundamental information regarding the mechanism of muscle adaptation to exercise. For instance, determining the molecular mechanism underlying the low-glycogen training effect may lead to the development of novel treatments for diseases such as diabetes that result from altered muscle metabolic function. Before it can be successfully applied to the athletic situation, however, more questions need to be answered about the potential for negative outcomes, and the optimum way to integrate some specific train low sessions into the periodized training program. It may prove difficult to undertake the sophisticated studies needed to define the optimal protocols, just as it is difficult for sports scientists to educate athletes and coaches about the true interpretations and applications of their work.

References

1　Bernard C: Nouvelles recherches expérimentales sur les phénomènes glycogeniques du foie. Comptes Rendus Soc Biol 1858;2:1–7.

2　Stetten D Jr, Stetten MR: Glycogen metabolism. Physiol Rev 1960;40:505–537.

3　Parnas JK, Ostern P: Le Mechanisme de la glycogenolyse. Bull Soc Chim Biol 1936;18:1471–1492.

4　Cori GT, Cori CF: The kinetics of the enzymatic synthesis of glycogen from glucose-1-phosphate. J Biol Chem 1940;135:733–756.

5　Bergstrom J, Hermansen L, Hultman E, et al: Diet, muscle glycogen and physical performance. Acta Physiol Scand 1967;71:140–150.

6　Hultman E, Bergstrom J: Muscle glycogen synthesis in relation to diet studied in normal subjects. Acta Med Scand 1967;182:109–117.

7　Bergstrom J, Hultman E: Synthesis of muscle glycogen in man after glucose and fructose infusion. Acta Med Scand 1967;182:93–107.

8　Johnston JD, Schlader ZJ, Mickleborough TD, et al: Nutritional considerations for the endurance athlete. Glycogen replenishment following intense exercise. Agrofood Industry Hi-Tech 2007;18:XI–XIV.

9 Blomstrand E, Saltin B: Effect of muscle glycogen on glucose, lactate and amino acid metabolism during exercise and recovery in human subjects. J Physiol 1999;514: 293–302.

10 Steensberg A, van Hall G, Keller C, et al: Muscle glycogen content and glucose uptake during exercise in humans influence of prior exercise and dietary manipulation. J Physiol 2002;541:273–281.

11 Hansen AK, Fischer CP, Plomgaard P, et al: Skeletal muscle adaptation. Training twice every second day vs. training once daily. J Appl Physiol 2005;98:93–99.

12 Hulston CJ, Venables MC, Mann CH, et al: Training with low muscle glycogen enhances fat metabolism in well-trained cyclists. Med Sci Sports Exerc 2010;42:2046–2055.

13 Yeo WK, Paton CD, Garnham AP, et al: Skeletal muscle adaptation and performance responses to once a day versus twice every second day endurance training regimens. J Appl Physiol 2008;105:1462–1470.

14 Widegren U, Jiang XJ, Krook A, et al: Divergent effects of exercise on metabolic and mitogenic signaling pathways in human skeletal muscle. FASEB J 1998;12:1379–1389.

15 Akimoto T, Sorg BS, Yan Z: Real-time imaging of peroxisome proliferator-activated receptor-gamma coactivator-1alpha promoter activity in skeletal muscles of living mice. Am J Physiol Cell Physiol 2004;287:C790–C796.

16 Miura S, Kawanaka K, Kai Y, et al: An increase in murine skeletal muscle PGC-1α mRNA in response to exercise is mediated by β-adrenergic receptor activation. Endocrinology 2007;148:3441–3448.

17 Chinsomboon J, Ruas J, Gupta RK, et al: The transcriptional coactivator PGC-1alpha mediates exercise-induced angiogenesis in skeletal muscle. Proc Natl Acad Sci USA 2009;106:21401–21406.

18 Mortensen OH, Plomgaard P, Fischer CP, et al: PGC-1beta is downregulated by training in human skeletal muscle. No effect of training twice every second day vs. once daily on expression of the PGC-1 family. J Appl Physiol 2007;103:1536–1542.

19 Robinson MM, Richards JC, Hickey MS, et al: Acute β-adrenergic stimulation does not alter mitochondrial protein synthesis or markers of mitochondrial biogenesis in adult men. Am J Physiol Regul Integr Comp Physiol 2010;298:R25–R33.

20 Towler MC, Hardie DG: AMP-activated protein kinase in metabolic control and insulin signaling. Circ Res 2007;100:328–341.

21 Zong H, Ren JM, Young LH, et al: AMP kinase is required for mitochondrial biogenesis in skeletal muscle in response to chronic energy deprivation. Proc Natl Acad Sci USA 2002;99:15983–15987.

22 Viollet B, Andreelli F, Jorgensen SB, et al: The AMP-activated protein kinase alpha2 catalytic subunit controls whole-body insulin sensitivity. J Clin Invest 2003;111:91–98.

23 Sakamoto K, McCarthy A, Smith D, et al: Deficiency of LKB1 in skeletal muscle prevents AMPK activation and glucose uptake during contraction. EMBO J 2005;24:1810–1820.

24 Wojtaszewski JF, MacDonald C, Nielsen JN, et al: Regulation of 5′AMP-activated protein kinase activity and substrate utilization in exercising human skeletal muscle. Am J Physiol Endocrinol Metab 2003;284:E813–E822.

25 Akerstrom TC, Birk JB, Klein DK, et al: Oral glucose ingestion attenuates exercise-induced activation of 5′-AMP-activated protein kinase in human skeletal muscle. Biochem Biophys Res Commun 2006;342:949–955.

26 Lee-Young RS, Palmer MJ, Linden KC, et al: Carbohydrate ingestion does not alter skeletal muscle AMPK signaling during exercise in humans. Am J Physiol Endocrinol Metab 2006;291:E566–E573.

27 McBride A, Ghilagaber S, Nikolaev A, Hardie DG: The glycogen-binding domain on the AMPK beta subunit allows the kinase to act as a glycogen sensor. Cell Metab 2009;7;9:23–34.

28 Steinberg GR, Watt MJ, McGee SL, et al: Reduced glycogen availability is associated with increased AMPKalpha2 activity, nuclear AMPKalpha2 protein abundance, and GLUT4 mRNA expression in contracting human skeletal muscle. Appl Physiol Nutr Metab 2006;31:302–312.

29 McGee SL, Sparling D, Olson AL, et al: Exercise increases MEF2- and GEF DNA-binding activity in human skeletal muscle. FASEB J 2006;20:348–349.

30 Narkar VA, Downes M, Yu RT, et al: AMPK and PPARdelta agonists are exercise mimetics. Cell 2008;134:405–415.

31 Bussau VA, Fairchild TJ, Rao A, et al: Carbohydrate loading in human muscle: an improved 1 day protocol. Eur J Appl Physiol 2002;87:290–295.

32 Burke LM: Fueling strategies to optimize performance: training high or training low? Scand J Med Sci Sports 2010;20(suppl 2): 48–58.

33 Hawley JA, Burke LM: Carbohydrate availability and training adaptation: effects on cell metabolism. Exerc Sport Sci Rev 2010;38:152–160.

34 Morton JP, Croft L, Bartlett JD, et al: Reduced carbohydrate availability does not modulate training-induced heat shock protein adaptations but does upregulate oxidative enzyme activity in human skeletal muscle. J Appl Physiol 2009;106:1513–1521.

35 Creer A, Gallagher P, Slivka D, et al: Influence of muscle glycogen availability on ERK1/2 and Akt signaling after resistance exercise in human skeletal muscle. J Appl Physiol 2005;99:950–956.

36 Hopkins WG, Hawley JA, Burke LM: Design and analysis of research on sport performance enhancement. Med Sci Sports Exerc 1999;31:472–485.

37 Rodriguez NR, Di Marco NM, Langley S, et al: American College of Sports Medicine position stand. Nutrition and athletic performance. Med Sci Sports Exerc 2009;41: 709–731.

38 Stellingwerff T, Spriet LL, Watt MJ, et al: Decreased PDH activation and glycogenolysis during exercise following fat adaptation with carbohydrate restoration. Am J Physiol Endocrinol Metab 2006;290:E380–E388.

39 Havemann L, West SJ, Goedecke JH, et al: Fat adaptation followed by carbohydrate loading compromises high-intensity sprint performance. J Appl Physiol 2006;100:194–202.

40 Gleeson M, Nieman DC, Pedersen BK: Exercise, nutrition and immune function. J Sports Sci 2004;22:115–122.

41 Brouns F, Saris WHM, Ten Hoor F: Nutrition as a factor in the prevention of injuries in recreational and competitive downhill skiing. J Sports Med 1986;26:85–91.

42 Petibois C, Cazorla G, Poortmans JR et al: Biochemical aspects of overtraining in endurance sports: the metabolism alteration process syndrome. Sports Med 2003;33:83–94.

Discussion

Dr. Burke: The opportunity to work with you on this topic has been interesting because we come to it from different perspectives. If I can use a gross generalization: I come from a world where success is measured in terms of gold medals, while the academic world is driven by 'publish or perish'. So, while we can appreciate each other's work, it doesn't always mean we are pursuing the same ends or speaking the same language. The new techniques in molecular biology provide fascinating insights into what happens when a stimulus is applied acutely or repeatedly to the muscle, but I am interested in intact humans and the application of a variety of changing stimuli. How do we take the 'black and white' details of these complex molecular insights into my world? How do we set up a molecular model with all the variables associated with the periodized training and nutrition programs undertaken by real-life athletes? And how can we decide if the outcomes make a difference to sports performance, or even on systems outside the muscle?

Dr. Baar: What I did here is talk exclusively about muscle. There is no reason that you need to periodize for strength as far as the muscle is concerned. But what happens outside the muscle, in the connective tissue, is much different from what is happening in muscle, and there is a much slower adaptation. The same thing is true in an endurance individual, where the base phase is the perfect time to do low glycogen training to maximize endurance capacity. But as you increase the speed, using more high-quality sessions, you are actually decreasing the focus on the muscular component and increasing the stress on the connective tissue system. Although I didn't talk about it, we should consider how these things interact. We know that myostatin has a negative effect on muscle mass, but it has a very positive effect on the connective tissue. If you talk to Pfizer, they think the best thing you can do for an old person is to get rid of myostatin but I think that's the worst thing to do, because they will have a bigger muscle but it will weaken the connective tissue. It is very similar to when people started using steroids without growth hormone or anything to help the connective tissue. The steroids targeted skeletal muscle exclusively, the connective tissue didn't improve at all, and the rate of injury went through the roof.

In the discussion here, we are somewhat blinded because we focused on the muscle and specifically metabolism within the muscle. When you step back and you look at the whole organism, it's much more difficult because you're trying to integrate a signal that is positive for the skeletal muscle but perhaps negative for other issues. As far as low glycogen training is concerned, having only looked at muscle, it's very difficult for me to say that there is a certain training benefit or that there is one molecule that is going to be the key. But I think it would be impossible to look only at the whole organism with an intervention as complex as exercise and try to make significant scientific advances. You do that with performance. But to actually understand the mechanism of how performance is improved, I don't think that's possible using only the whole organism.

If we came back to talk about connective tissue, we would have a whole different group of things to consider or a whole different way to look at our intervention. With a positive effect on skeletal muscle, and a negative effect on connective tissue, we need to find the best balance to get optimal performance. That's what you are trying to do with periodization. For example, we believe that the best thing we can do for muscle performance is to train at a high cadence so if you are a runner train at a high speed. However, that is the worst thing you can do for the connective tissue because it's going to be extremely damaging, especially if there is not enough recovery time, since connective tissue recovers more slowly. As a result, the runners will periodize their workouts to try to balance the positives for skeletal muscle with the negatives for connective tissue to come up with the best combination of those two for performance. When we boil down low glycogen training and look at only the skeletal muscle, I can say that PPARs are playing a role – not necessarily, the only thing that is happening – that seems to be positive in certain situations. Whether the PPARs are going to be positive in all the cell types in the body, or whether they will have a negative effect on other tissues, I can't tell you just by looking at the muscle.

Dr. Zemel: It's very difficult to manipulate glycogen without changing everything else as well, including fatty acid concentrations. You also linked fatty acids with PPARs, so how much do you think the findings of your work have to do with low glycogen and how much do they have to do with fatty acids?

Dr. Baar: Right now I would say that, at least on the PPAR side, the adaptation that we see for enzymes involved with fatty acid uptake and oxidation does not have anything to do with the low glycogen directly. We are manipulating glycogen because that's what we can control, but in the background the fat is going up and compensating. We end up with a situation where we can acutely do what the people who do fat manipulation (increased dietary fat) do over a longer term. In either case, PPAR is activated and that's one of the key adaptations. So all we are doing is instead of having to go through a week or a number of days of chronic changes to the diet, in a single day with the two sessions we are activating the same transcription factor that probably underlies the fat adaptation response. So, at least as far as PPAR activation is concerned, I think that it's all dependent on the fat.

Dr. Zemel: What were the fatty acid concentrations in your animal work, and is this realistically achievable in humans?

Dr. Baar: Our cell culture work uses 250 μM fatty acids because we are trying to reach a high physiological level. Of course, at the moment, this is a single fatty acid, since we perform our experiments in a serum-free medium and add only one fatty acid each time. In the future, we will combine the best individual fatty acids to see whether there is an additive effect. We can also test other metabolites that seem to have a positive effect in parallel. We have already done it with the nutraceutical ECGC because it was supposed to have a similar effect to low glycogen training, but we don't see any effect of ECGC in isolated muscle. Rather, we think there is a whole body effect where ECGC causes the release of fat from the adipose which trickles down to the muscle, resulting in more delivery of fatty acids, and the same increase in PPAR activity that we see with the low-glycogen training.

Dr. van Loon: I would like to explore your work on the anaplerotic amino acids. We have some overlapping data, but there are all sorts of striking differences that may be related to timing and dose. If we look at leucine, we see something similar to what you see: an increase in PGC1α, an increase in mitochondrial biogenesis and an increase in fat oxidation, but it takes some time – it's a structure-independent effect. When we do the same thing with C2C12 myotubes and the other branch chain amino acids, we see absolutely nothing when using a low-glucose medium.

Dr. Baar: We don't see a great effect in a low- or normal-glucose environment, but we see anaplerotic effects when we give a carbohydrate or high-fat challenge. For example, if we increase the fatty acid or the sugar content of the media we would normally see an inhibition of metabolic function, whereas if at the same time you give an anaplerotic amino acid you reverse that entirely. That's how we have done the experiments: we have given pyruvate or glucose or fructose, and then we supplement so you have got two entry points to the TCA cycle.

We have done everything from 0.5 to 50 mM. The 50 mM has a huge effect, but this is way outside the physiological range. However, we still get the effects within the physiological range – a 0.5 mM range. Of course, the glucose within the medium will decline over time. We refresh the medium every 12 h to try to get around the normal decline in substrate and build up of waste, since it is also important to remember that the cells are producing a lot of lactate and lactate accumulation may cause adaptations as well.

Dr. van Loon: Are the effects of using high glucose and any of the anaplerotic amino acids fairly rapid?

Dr. Baar: The PGC1α transcriptional data that I showed are the effects of 3 h of treatment, so relatively rapid. We have done 3 days of treatment and see increases in oxygen consumption rate, but these effects take longer because they represent wholesale changes within the muscle cells.

Dr. Maughan: You talked about the historical developments in the understanding of glycogen metabolism. You said, initially people thought it was broken down to glucose, but then they realized that it was glucose phosphate. Of course, about 10% is liberated as free glucose, and if you do high-intensity exercise with high glycogen content, you have the unique situation of very high glycolysis rates that will achieve very high intracellular free glucose. What's the role of that free glucose in all of these things?

Dr. Baar: I don't know about the free glucose per se, but the position of those free glucose moieties is very interesting and may be important. If you look at proteins like AMP kinase that have glycogen-binding domains, they seem to have a preference for the branch points, and it's specifically the branch points that lead to increased arborization. People like Graham Hardie think that as glycogen is broken down, cleavage of the branch point sugars results in a signal that there is a serious decrease in glycogen. The proteins that bind to these sites, specifically AMP kinase and glycogen synthase, are released and activated and they serve to put a brake on metabolic processes in the muscle: decreasing anabolic and increasing catabolic processes. So whether it's a signal and whether free glucose could be a measure of the activation of proteins that have a glycogen binding domain, I don't know but it is an interesting observation.

Dr. Spriet: In your cell work, do you include insulin? Most people argue that the initial upregulation of PDK4 that occurs whenever you limit the carbohydrate source is due to low levels of insulin.

Dr. Baar: The data that I presented here were mainly the pyruvate data where the effects occur independent of insulin. When we use glucose or fructose for the carbon overload, we add a small amount of insulin.

Dr. Spriet: With the 'two a day training' in humans, you are putting quite a bit of stock on the increase in catecholamines associated with low glycogen. But is that something that persists day after day or does it decrease as you continue the training?

Dr. Hawley: We haven't measured that in our studies but it's a good question – do you adapt to it or does it just drop? I suspect it drops.

Dr. Spriet: It's a strange thing because with very high-intensity exercise you get very high epinephrine levels, and yet your ability to mobilize fat either from adipose tissue or the muscle seems to be limited, indicating that something else is overriding it. Epinephrine levels are higher when working at 85% versus 60% of maximal aerobic capacity, yet you don't get as much free fatty acids out of the adipose tissue, and you don't break down as much intramuscular fat. So, in spite of those signals being present, they are overridden by other regulators.

Dr. Baar: The data of Romijn and colleagues suggest that the lack of release of fatty acids from the fat is due to constriction of the blood vessels to the adipose tissue and that if you increase circulating fatty acids you can oxidize approximately 30% more fatty acids.

Dr. Spriet: Yes, the lipolytic rate stays up in adipose tissue, and interestingly inside the muscle the high levels of AMPK are actually overriding the effects of contraction and the effects of the epinephrine at higher exercise intensities.

Dr. Baar: It's a possibility. Thinking back to some of the early work that Larry Oscai did with HSL and lipoprotein lipase in skeletal muscle during exercise and following training, I wonder whether part of the response and a component of improving fat oxidation is actually to increase the amount and the activity of these lipases. That could have a positive effect on being able to import more triglyceride from the circulation and free more triglyceride out of the intramuscular stores.

Dr. Spriet: When you measure the amount of HSL in the 'a' or active form, it's definitely down at higher exercise intensities. However, little work has been done in muscle on the newly discovered enzyme, adipose tissue triacylglycerol lipase (ATGL).

Dr. Baar: Again, that suggests that HSL and ATGL could be a key limitation in this situation. Increasing HSL or ATGL could increase the amount of fat that you could oxidize at a high intensity, but I don't know.

Dr. van Loon: It has previously been reported that free fatty acid concentrations in the cytosol increase during high intensity exercise, so free intracellular free fatty acid availability is unlikely to be a limitation to fat oxidation.

Dr. Baar: If there is an increase in free fatty acids within the cytosol at high intensity, you would expect that they either have a signaling role, which is entirely possible, or that there is another limitation, and the obvious limitation is CPT1. Work from Clinton Bruce from Australia has shown that when they increase CPT1 in muscle, by overexpression, they see a positive effect on fatty acid oxidation. This would suggest that CPT1 does limit fat oxidation as well. Interestingly, CPT1 and HSL levels are both transcriptionally controlled by PPARs.

Of course, overexpression experiments can cause many side effects. However, the Bruce experiment was a transient overexpression using electroporation in adult muscle, so fewer side effects would occur. If we view training through the lens of molecular biology, what we are trying to do is get the body to produce more of the key proteins responsible for adaptation: a transient overexpression if you will. By repeating this training stimulus, we are trying to establish a new steady state where we have increased proteins like HSL and CPT1 and this will result in greater fat oxidation.

Dr. Hoppeler: You mentioned that it's not only muscle tissue but connective tissue – and, of course, capillaries are very important. Do you have any comments on these alternate promoters of PGC1α and the capillary vessel?

Dr. Baar: Zoltan Arany's work showed quite nicely that the capillarization is dependent on PGC1α and the estrogen receptor-related (ERR) α-protein. ERRα is one of the proteins that PGC1α coactivates. If I remember correctly, his group showed that neither the PGC1α muscle-specific knockout nor the ERRα knockout mice show angiogenesis following exercise. That would indicate to me that the angiogenic response is dependent on PGC1α. So, PGC1α plays a role in angiogenesis, but there may be other factors involved as well including angiogenic growth factors. How those are influenced by nutrient interventions has yet to be determined.

Dr. Gibala: My bias is that anaplerosis, or at least the exercise-induced expansion of the TCA cycle intermediate pool during exercise, has absolutely nothing to do with the regulation of oxidative metabolism in humans. We have conducted a number of studies where we tried to manipulate TCA cycle intermediates during exercise but found no effect on performance or markers of oxidative metabolism. How do you measure anaplerosis in your studies, and how does it impact TCA cycle flux? Do you measure TCA cycle intermediates?

Dr. Baar: The way we have done this is using a Seahorse metabolic flux machine, and we use acetate as a measure of TCA flux. We don't have the capacity to measure the TCA intermediates. We add acetate and look to see what happens to oxygen consumption. If TCA flux is higher, there is a bigger increase in oxygen consumption when we give acetate. The experiments involve treating muscle cells for 3 days with the anaplerotic amino acids or non-anaplerotic amino acids and then measuring the change in acetate flux.

Dr. Gibala: Is it due to the increase in the intermediates, or could they be going out through cataplerosis and then entering back into the cycle at the level of the acetyl-CoA, so it's just additional substrate.

Dr. Baar: We don't think it is additional substrate, because what we see in glycolytic overload is a decrease in ATP consumption. We see an increase in fatty acid oxidation enzymes but no increase in fat uptake or oxidation even though PDH phosphorylation is high. So, it doesn't look to us like providing more acetyl-CoA would have a positive effect. We have also used anaplerotic amino acids that enter the TCA cycle at different points, and it seems like the amino acids that enter at SDH have the strongest effect. So, to us this suggests that having substrates enter the TCA cycle at more than one point can overcome a block in acetyl-CoA entry. The result is an increase in flux through the TCA cycle.

That brings up the possibility that what exercise does is increase the flux through the TCA cycle, and that is one of the signals to increase PGC1α. When we looked at all of the standard candidates to signal to PGC1α, not a single one of them was changing. But we know that there is more flux and this creates a rapid change in PGC1α, and so all we can conclude is that the flux itself increases PGC1α. In fact, it could be that anything that increases TCA flux increases PGC1α and improves muscle metabolism, whereas anything that decreases flux leads to insulin resistance and metabolic disease. The difference between your work and ours is that in our systems there was metabolic overload, whereas you looked at exercising people in a normal metabolic state. We see this a lot, if you have a deficiency and you supplement there is a positive effect, but the same positive effect is not seen when you give the same supplement to a complete system. So, that's what we have in the glycolytic or fat overload situation: we have a diseased system. When we give the anaplerotic amino acids in these 'disease' states, we have a beneficial effect, whereas in the normal situation this would not be the case.

Dr. Hawley: I know that the human model I am using is a 'dirty model', and it seems like your reductionist approach is very good to tease out mechanisms, but to bring it back to the practical side, we use a different model from the Hansen studies. We get our guys to exercise maximally at the highest intensity possible, so presumably catecholamines and other hormones are high, but the problem is that our subjects feel terrible and train at a lower intensity. So, we are now addressing in a series of studies whether we can alleviate some of the central and peripheral fatigue by giving them caffeine or a little bit of glucose. This might allow subjects to feel better and train with low glycogen at a higher intensity. We have preliminary data that caffeine supplementation partially rescues training capacity, but doesn't rescue up to the point of training with normal glycogen. The further question to ask is whether that level of rescue can change the overall performance outcome from training with low glycogen.

Dr. Baar: That will be the key aspect. The other issue with caffeine is that you are looking at something that might also affect calcium signaling, which might have an additional effect. All you have to do is to get around a lot of this central limitation or the negative feelings of fatigue, is to fool the brain into thinking that it will be getting sugars soon. Carter and colleagues showed that rinsing the mouth with a sugar drink improves performance. So, I think the more precise way might be give a mouth wash with a sweet solution to give them a performance boost without a metabolic interference.

Dr. Burke: It's great to see what's happening at the level of the muscle, but to me the functional outcome is what's most important. So even if caffeine adds some additional factors to the mixture, at the end of the day if the athlete who trains with caffeine can perform better, do we really care?

Dr. Baar: The reason we need to understand the mechanism is so we can maximize it. If I know what I want to maximize in the muscle, I can produce a high throughput test to see which nutrients maximize it. For example, with the PPAR activation, I can test 40 compounds at a time and know the result in 9 h, whereas with an athlete you will have to train for 3–6 weeks before you know the effects of a single intervention. In order for you to go through all of the different interventions, it would take much longer, and that's the difference. If you can boil it down to a very basic thing; if you understand which molecules to look at, you can quickly look at thousands of compounds. This is the power of molecular biology. If a few look really good in the lab, we can then move to translate those to the athlete. This is what I think is lost in the translation from people who are talking about the molecules to the people who are really only focused on performance. We need to meet in the middle. I can identify a handful of foods, fats, sugars, etc. that maximize the response in the lab, and then it is up to the performance scientist to determine whether any of these are beneficial to performance.

Dr. Burke: I guess that's the bottom line. We need to work together because you can efficiently identify what could be important, getting it to the point where I can take over and do the performance studies. By ourselves, we haven't got the complete picture. I think that's a problem at the moment because some people, even educated athletes and coaches with access to the internet, can go straight to the molecular work and consider this a proxy for performance. We need to keep pushing the value of the performance study to make sure that it actually translates.

Maughan RJ, Burke LM (eds): Sports Nutrition: More Than Just Calories – Triggers for Adaptation.
Nestlé Nutr Inst Workshop Ser, vol 69, pp 39–58,
Nestec Ltd., Vevey/S. Karger AG., Basel, © 2011

Metabolic Regulation of Fat Use during Exercise and in Recovery

Lawrence L. Spriet

Department of Human Health and Nutritional Science, University of Guelph, Guelph, ON, Canada

Abstract

Fat is an important fuel for exercise but plays a secondary role to carbohydrate (CHO). Increasing fat use during exercise can decrease the reliance on CHO and spare CHO for later in training sessions or competitions that depend on CHO for success. The pathways that metabolize and oxidize fat are activated more slowly than CHO at the onset of exercise and reach a maximum at moderate exercise intensities. As exercise intensity increases to $\sim75\%$ VO_{2max} and beyond, fat metabolism is inhibited: using CHO will increase the amount of energy produced per liter of oxygen consumed. The capacity for fat use during exercise is increased by aerobic training and the dietary combination of little or no CHO intake and high fat intake. Fat oxidation is very dependent on the mitochondrial volume of muscle but other key sites of regulation include release of fat from storage forms and fat transport across plasma and mitochondrial membranes. This chapter examines the control of fat metabolism during moderate and intense exercise with an emphasis on human findings and the adaptations that occur with aerobic training and other acute nutritional manipulations. Recent work using molecular and cellular compartmentalization techniques have advanced the knowledge in this area.

Introduction

Work in the early 1900s demonstrated that both fat and carbohydrate (CHO) could be used as fuel for muscular contractions and that the amount of fat and CHO used depended on several factors [1]. The preceding diet was the main factor during short-duration aerobic exercise of low to moderate intensity. As exercise intensity increased, the proportion of fat oxidation decreased, and CHO oxidation increased such that fat use was virtually absent at 100% VO_{2max}. While CHO can provide all the substrate required for exercise at $\sim$100% VO_{2max}, fat can

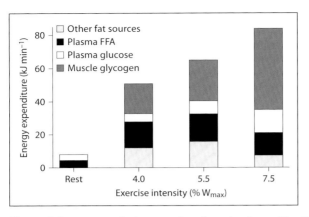

Fig. 1. Substrate use during exercise of varying intensities [6].

only provide substrate at a rate to sustain ~60–75% VO_{2max} when CHO availability is severely restricted. However, during prolonged moderate-intensity exercise, the relative fat contribution increases due to the increasing availability of plasma free fatty acid (FFA) and decreasing CHO stores. Later studies used more direct experimental approaches to demonstrate the importance of plasma FFA and fat derived from stores inside the muscle (IMTG) as substrates for oxidation during exercise and showed that the absolute amount of fat oxidized was largely a function of the mitochondrial volume of the contracting musculature [2–4].

The pathways that mobilize and deliver fat to the mitochondria are not activated as quickly as CHO metabolism at the onset of exercise, and fat oxidation is inhibited as exercise intensity approaches ~75–85% VO_{2max} [5, 6] (fig. 1). While important adaptations occur with exercise training, human skeletal muscle is not engineered to maximize fat use during intense aerobic exercise. Maximal fat oxidation occurs at ~60–65% VO_{2max}, whereas many athletic and sports situations take place at >80% VO_{2max}.

Overview of the Regulation of Fat Metabolism

To understand the potential importance of exercise training and sports nutrition to trigger adaptations in fat metabolism that may lead to improved exercise performance, we need to understand the regulation of fat metabolism. Until recently, knowledge in this area lagged far behind that of CHO metabolism, but new research has revealed many of the sites of control in adipose tissue and skeletal muscle.

Potential control points that regulate fat metabolism in skeletal muscle during aerobic exercise include: (1) adipose tissue lipolysis, FFA release from

Spriet

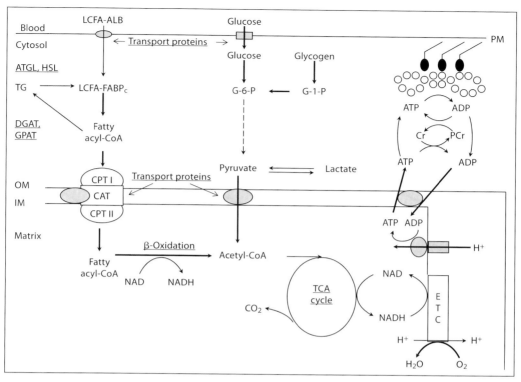

Fig. 2. Schematic overview of fat metabolism in skeletal muscle. PM = Plasma membrane; OM, IM = outer and inner mitochondrial membranes; ALB = albumin; LCFA = long-chain fatty acid; GPAT = glycerol-phosphate acyltransferase; DGAT = diacylglycerol acyltransferase; CAT = carnitine-acylcarnitine translocase; NAD^+, NADH = oxidized and reduced nicotinamide adenine dinucleotide; G-6-P, G-1-P = glucose 6- and 1-phosphate; PCr = phosphocreatine; Cr = creatine; TCA = tricarboxylic acid; ETC = electron transport chain. Shaded circles and boxes depict transport proteins.

adipose tissue, and delivery to the muscle, (2) FFA transport across the muscle membrane, (3) binding and transport of FFA in the cytoplasm, (4) IMTG lipolysis, (5) FFA transport across the mitochondrial membranes, and possibly (6) metabolism in the β-oxidation pathway (fig. 2). Manipulation of the skeletal muscle mitochondrial volume, which determines the overall capacity to oxidize fat, might also be considered an overarching control point.

Long-chain FFA derived from adipose tissue are a major source of fat for the working muscle during exercise. The degradation of FFA from adipose tissue triacylglycerol (TG) and the release and removal of FFA from adipose tissue are regulated processes, and much work has examined the control of the regulatory enzymes, hormone-sensitive lipase (HSL) and the newly discovered adipose tissue triglyceride lipase (ATGL) [7]. A constant supply of albumin in the blood perfusing adipose tissue is also required to allow the FFAs to bind to albumin, as transport of FFA in the blood and muscle cells requires a protein chaperone. Bulk transport of FFA to the muscle ([FFA] × blood flow) also plays a role in the uptake of FFA by muscle. A reduction in the ability to move newly released FFA out of the adipose tissue and into the blood appears to be a major reason for the lack of an increase in plasma [FFA] during exercise at ~80% vs. 40–60% VO_{2max} as the lipolytic rate does not decrease at the higher power output [5]. Important questions in this area include how we speed up these processes of fat mobilization at the onset of exercise and maintain an adequate blood flow to this tissue during intense aerobic exercise.

Recent evidence suggests that the majority of the FFAs entering muscle cells are transported or assisted across the muscle membrane by transport proteins, most notably the fatty acid translocase protein (FAT/CD36), the plasma membrane fatty acid-binding protein ($FABP_{pm}$), and members of the fatty acid transport protein family [8, 9]. FAT/CD36 also translocates to the plasma membrane during 2 h of cycling at 60% VO_{2max} to facilitate FFA movement into the cell [unpubl. obs.]. It is not clear what occurs during more intense exercise, and whether there may actually be a decrease in membrane fat transport proteins. Once inside the muscle, FFAs are bound to cytoplasmic FABP ($FABP_c$). The FFA destined for storage as IMTG or for oxidation in the mitochondria must first be 'activated' by coupling to coenzyme A (CoA) through the activity of fatty acyl-CoA synthase.

A second major source of fat is via the release of FFA from IMTG. The first events in regulating muscle lipolysis are activation of the TG lipases, including muscle versions of ATGL and HSL. Additional regulatory steps appear to include movement of the ATGL-HSL complex to the lipid droplet, and penetration of a protective perilipin-like protein layer around the lipid droplet. Lipid droplets are found in close proximity to mitochondria, and it is likely that the regulatory proteins/enzymes involved in activating fat for storage or oxidation, transport into the mitochondria, TG synthesis, and TG degradation are all in close contact [4]. These enzymes appear to be sensitive to both hormonal and contractile stimuli during exercise, and IMTG provides an important energy source during moderate intensity exercise [10, 11]. The activity of HSL actually decreases during intense aerobic exercise, which may be the result of increased AMP kinase (AMPK) activity and contribute to a decrease in IMTG use [11]. However, current understanding of the coordinated regulation of ATGL and HSL during exercise in human skeletal muscle is rudimentary. Lastly, there is also evidence to suggest that increasing plasma FFA levels and uptake of FFA into the cell decreases the reliance on IMTG during moderate exercise lasting 2–4 h [12].

For oxidation to occur, cytoplasmic $FABP_c$-FFA, whether derived from outside the cell (plasma FFA) or inside muscle (IMTG), must be transported to the outer mitochondrial membrane. It is then activated with CoA, if not already activated, and converted to fatty acyl carnitine by carnitine palmitoyltransferase I (CPT I). This compound is moved across the mitochondrial membranes via a translocase, while carnitine moves in the opposite direction. Recent evidence also suggests that the transfer of fatty acyl carnitine across the membranes is aided in some unidentified manner by the fat transport protein FAT/CD36, and that this protein translocates to the mitochondrial membranes during 2 h of moderate-intensity exercise [13]. Inside the mitochondria, carnitine is removed, and the CoA is rebound to the long-chain fatty acid by the enzyme CPT II.

The level of free carnitine may inhibit mitochondrial FFA uptake during intense exercise as it is a substrate for the CPT I reaction [14]. Muscle carnitine content decreases as a function of increasing exercise intensity, and a low free carnitine level could limit FFA transport into the mitochondria and FFA oxidation during intense exercise when glycolytic flux is high. It is not currently known how much free carnitine is needed in the cytoplasm to maintain CPT I-mediated FFA transport into the mitochondria. However, the highest rates of FFA oxidation occur when the carnitine levels are already substantially lower than resting levels and carnitine is not consumed in the transport process, but recycled back into the cytoplasm. In addition, when fat availability in the blood is artificially increased during intense exercise (~80% VO_{2max}) the muscle oxidizes more fat, suggesting that the level of muscle carnitine is not limiting for fat oxidation at intense power outputs [15]. Collectively, these factors make it unlikely that free carnitine availability limits FFA oxidation during intense exercise, but Stephens et al. [14] have been able to increase muscle carnitine levels by a modest 15% with a 5-hour infusion of carnitine and insulin. This resulted in an apparent increase in fat oxidation, but the results are confounded by the fact that the hyperinsulinemia would increase the content of muscle membrane and mitochondrial fat transport proteins, which may also contribute to increased fat oxidation. In conclusion, no experimental model has been able to conclusively test whether there is a causal relationship between increasing muscle carnitine levels and increased fat oxidation during intense exercise.

A second possible explanation for the decreased reliance on fat at higher power outputs involves the inhibition of CPT I activity. Studies on mitochondria isolated from resting human skeletal muscle reported that decreases in pH from 7 to 6.8, typical of the cellular changes when moving from moderate to intense aerobic exercise, caused large reductions in CPT I activity [16].

Once inside the mitochondria, fatty acyl-CoA molecules are metabolized in the β-oxidation pathway to produce acetyl-CoA and reducing equivalents (NADH, $FADH_2$). There is currently no evidence that the enzymes of the β-oxidation pathway are externally regulated, suggesting that regulation is simply a function of the availability of pathway substrates (fatty acyl-CoA, NAD^+, FAD, and free CoA) and products (NADH, $FADH_2$, and acetyl-CoA). The most effective way to change the control or increase the capacity of the β-oxidation pathway is to increase the mitochondrial content, as occurs with exercise training. The maximal activity of β-hydroxyacyl-CoA dehydrogenase (β-HAD), a representative enzyme in the β-oxidation pathway, is commonly used to assess the magnitude of the adaptation to training, as discussed below.

Exercise Training Increases Fat Oxidation during Exercise

Holloszy [17] and Holloszy and Coyle [18] in the late 1960s and early 1970s demonstrated the remarkable plasticity of rat skeletal muscle, including the ability to increase the mitochondrial volume and the production of energy from fat and CHO. These landmark studies spawned the field of exercise-induced mitochondrial biogenesis, and additional work quickly confirmed these findings in human skeletal muscle [4, 19]. Work in this area continues to be at the forefront of research today as investigators revisit the early training studies with new and powerful molecular tools in an attempt to understand how skeletal muscle mitochondrial biogenesis results from the cumulative effects of transient increases in mRNA transcripts encoding mitochondrial proteins after successive exercise sessions [20–22]. This process requires the coordinated expression of both nuclear and mitochondrial (mtDNA) genomes through factors dedicated to specific families of genes encoding distinct categories of mitochondrial proteins.

A greater mitochondrial volume following training is believed to include increases in the fat-metabolizing machinery, as representative enzymes of the major fat-metabolizing pathways (e.g. citrate synthase, CS, β-HAD and cytochrome c oxidase IV) are also increased [17, 23]. This provides the means for a greater capacity to produce NADH from fat, and hence more ATP in the electron transport chain. The net result of these changes is a greater reliance on fat as a fuel and improved metabolic control (i.e. matching ATP production to ATP hydrolysis via oxidative mechanisms) during the onset of exercise at moderate and high aerobic exercise intensities. This results in reductions of the signals (free [ADP] and [AMP]) that activate the major enzymes that metabolize CHO (glycogen phosphorylase, phosphofructokinase and pyruvate dehydrogenase) and a decreased reliance on CHO for energy production at any given submaximal power output [17, 24].

The increased capacity for fat oxidation also requires increased provision of fatty acids, and it is not surprising that training increases plasma membrane and mitochondrial FA transport proteins [25]. In addition, endurance training also increases the IMTG store [4, 26] and increases HSL activity in some studies. A recent study has also reported an increase in ATGL activity [27]. Collectively, these adaptations alter the pattern of fuel utilization during submaximal exercise whereby whole body rates of fat oxidation are increased, while the rate of CHO oxidation is decreased, principally through the sparing of muscle glycogen, at both the same absolute and relative work rates as before training.

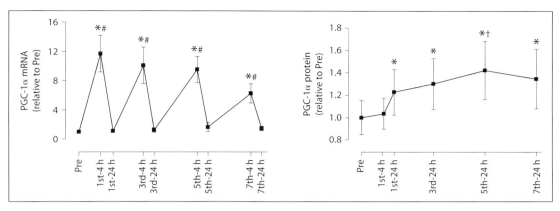

Fig. 3. Skeletal muscle PGC-1α and protein content throughout 2 weeks of high-intensity interval training. Values are means ± SE for 8–9 subjects. * $p < 0.05$, significantly different from Pre; # $p < 0.05$, significantly different from 1st-4 h; † $p < 0.05$, significantly different from 1st-24 h [22]. 1st, 3rd, 5th and 7th refer to the number of the exercise training session (each session was separated by 2 days). Measurements were made 4 and 24 h after an exercise session.

Recent molecular work has examined the time course of responses of mitochondrial biogenesis, mitochondrial fusion and fission proteins, and selected transcriptional and mitochondrial mRNAs and proteins in human muscle to seven sessions of intense interval training [23]. PGC-1α mRNA was increased >10-fold 4 h after the first session and returned to control within 24 h (fig. 3). This 'sawtooth' pattern continued until the 7th bout, with smaller increases after each bout. PGC-1α protein was increased 24 h after the first session (23%) and plateaued at +30–40% between bouts 3–7. Increases were observed in PPARα and -γ protein (1 session), PPARβ/δ mRNA and protein (5 sessions) and nuclear respiratory factor-2 protein (3 sessions), while no changes occurred in mitochondrial transcription factor A protein (fig. 5). CS and β-HAD mRNA were rapidly increased (1 session), followed by increases in CS and β-HAD activities (session 3), while changes in COX-IV mRNA (session 3) and protein (session 5) were more delayed (fig. 4). Training also increased mitochondrial fission proteins (fission protein-1, >2-fold; dynamin-related protein-1, 47%) and the fusion protein mitofusin-1 (35%) but not mitofusin-2. These data suggested that the training-induced increases in transcriptional and mitochondrial proteins resulted from the cumulative effects of transient bursts in their mRNAs and that training-induced mitochondrial biogenesis involved remodeling in addition to increased mitochondrial content. Importantly, it appears that the 'transcriptional capacity' of human muscle is extremely sensitive, being activated by one training bout. Recent work by Gibala [28] concluded that signaling through AMPK and p38 MAPK to PGC-1α may explain in part the metabolic remodeling induced by intense interval training, including mitochondrial biogenesis and an increased capacity for FFA oxidation.

Strategies to Increase Fat Oxidation in Already Well-Trained Athletes

A key area of interest is to find ways to increase fat oxidation in already well-trained athletes during exercise such that CHO use is curtailed or spared and is available for later in exercise in events where CHO availability is paramount for athletic success. Most of what we know regarding the ability to increase fat use has been derived from studies that used experimental manipulations to increase the plasma FFA availability without affecting many other processes. While many models have been used with varying success, including acute high-fat meals, short- and long-term high-fat diets, caffeine ingestion, fasting, and even prolonged dynamic exercise, the acute infusion of a lipid solution coupled with heparin administration has been most commonly and effectively used. This technique has the advantage of acutely (~30 min) increasing the plasma [FFA] without significant alterations in other substrates, metabolites and hormones [15, 29]. In contrast, dietary attempts to acutely increase the availability of endogenous FFA to the working muscles in humans immediately prior to or during exercise in an attempt to spare CHO have been largely unsuccessful as fat is not digested quickly. As a result, these practices are not used by athletes. Therefore, prolonged high-fat/low-CHO diets are required to alter the exogenous FFA availability and IMTG stores and spare CHO, as discussed in the following chapter. Lipid infusion with heparin injections is also not used by athletes, but these experiments demonstrated that starting moderate to intense exercise with elevated FFA levels (~1.0 vs. 0.3 mM) decreased glycogen use by ~50% in the initial 15 min of exercise and increased fat oxidation by ~15% with no change in exogenous glucose oxidation during 30 min of exercise [15, 29]. However, a decreased plasma FFA level is not the entire explanation for the decrease in fat oxidation with intense exercise. When plasma FFA availability during heavy exercise was increased to levels comparable to those observed during moderate intensity exercise, FFA oxidation was increased, but not fully restored [15]. This suggests that mechanisms within muscle as discussed previously and below also limit fatty acid oxidation at higher exercise intensities. Muscle measurements during exercise with elevated FFA revealed an attenuated rise in free ADP, AMP and P_i. This situation is similar to that found during steady-state exercise following aerobic training, where an increase in mitochondrial content and increased fat oxidation is believed to account for the attenuated insult to the energy state of the cell and reduction in CHO use. However, in the studies where FFA delivery was acutely altered, mitochondrial content was not altered, and therefore a key question is why the acute provision of exogenous fat provides a similar CHO-sparing effect to aerobic training.

Interestingly, caffeine ingestion also increases adipose tissue fat mobilization and skeletal muscle oxidation, but responses to this procedure vary between subjects, limiting what can be concluded on a group basis. When effective, caffeine appears to antagonize the normal inhibitory effects of adenosine on adipose

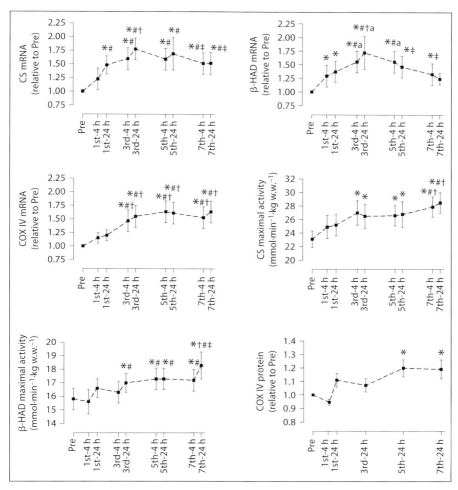

Fig. 4. Maximal activities and protein content of mitochondrial enzymes in skeletal muscle throughout 2 weeks of high-intensity interval training. Values are means ± SE for 9 subjects. * $p < 0.05$, significantly different from Pre; # $p < 0.05$, significantly different from 1st-4 h; † $p < 0.05$, significantly different from 1st-24 h; ‡ $p < 0.05$, significantly different from 3rd-24 h [22]. 1st, 3rd, 5th and 7th refer to the number of the exercise training session (each session was separated by 2 days). Measurements were made 4 and 24 h after an exercise session.

tissue lipolysis at rest, resulting in measurable increases in plasma FFA concentrations before exercise begins. The increased FFA delivery to and oxidation by the working muscles early in exercise appears to spare the use of muscle glycogen in some individuals [30]. However, the caffeine-induced increase in plasma FFA seen at rest does not increase adipose tissue lipolysis above the exercise effect, and no further glycogen sparing occurs beyond the first 10–20 min of exercise.

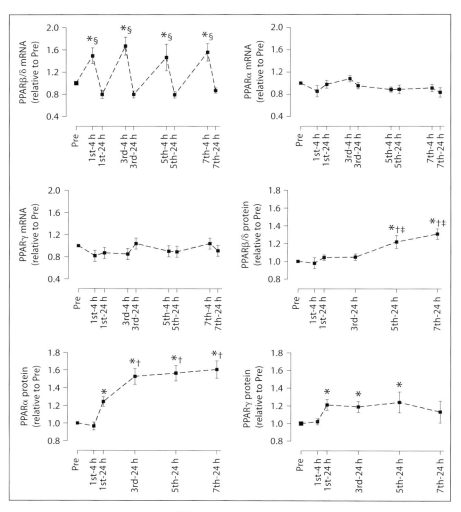

Fig. 5. Skeletal muscle PPARα, PPARβ/δ and PPARγ mRNA and protein content throughout 2 weeks of high-intensity interval training. Values are means ± SE for 8–9 subjects. * $p < 0.05$, significantly different from Pre; § $p < 0.05$, significantly different from all 24 h time points; † $p < 0.05$, significantly different from 1st-24 h; ‡ $p < 0.05$, significantly different from 3rd-24 h [22]. 1st, 3rd, 5th and 7th refer to the number of the exercise training session (each session was separated by 2 days). Measurements were made 4 and 24 h after an exercise session.

Another line of work examined the metabolism of long- and short-chain FFAs during moderate-intensity (~40% VO$_{2max}$) and heavy-intensity (~80% VO$_{2max}$) exercise, and while increasing the exercise intensity reduced long-chain FFA uptake and oxidation, the uptake and oxidation of medium-chain fatty acids (MCFA) was unaltered [31]. Since long-chain fatty acids rely on fat transport proteins to cross membranes and MCFAs are less dependent, this suggested an inhibitory effect of intense exercise and possibly of increased glycolytic flux on the oxidation of long-chain FFA. The location for this regulation likely involves plasma membrane transport and/or mitochondrial fat transport, both of which appear to be highly regulated for long-chain but not medium-chain FFAs.

Therefore, it would seem that the provision of medium-chain triacylglycerols to contracting skeletal muscle should augment the rate of FFA oxidation, as they are rapidly broken down in the stomach and duodenum and the MCFAs empty from the intestine into portal blood, are more soluble in plasma, and cross the muscle and mitochondrial membranes with less dependence on transport proteins. The same could be said for acetate, which freely enters the muscle and mitochondria and can be converted to acetyl-CoA in one step. Ingestion and infusion of these compounds produces accumulations in the blood at rest, and they are oxidized at rest. When exercise begins, these compounds continue to be oxidized in muscle and may account for up to 7–8% of the fuel used [32, 33]. However, they did not decrease the reliance on muscle glycogen to a significant amount to produce measurable glycogen sparing [33–35]. In the case of acetate, most studies have infused this compound as attempts to load the body through oral means are less effective. In the case of MCFA, the ability to ingest and move these fats into the bloodstream is dependent on the GI discomfort, and the ingestion of a tolerable amount (10 g/h) does not spare muscle glycogen or alter the patterns of fuel oxidation in muscle during exercise [34].

Strategies to increase fat oxidation in well-trained athletes at intense aerobic intensities need to elevate plasma FFA levels and target the key sites of fat metabolism and oxidation within the muscle itself. Nutritional schemes that have attempted to provide more FFA in the diet or increase adipose tissue lipolysis have been largely unsuccessful. Attempts to target the muscle and increase fat oxidation at high aerobic power outputs need to overcome what appears to be inherent or native mechanisms that decrease the reliance on fat and increase the reliance on CHO as a substrate.

Fat Metabolism during Recovery

As soon as an exercise training session or competition ends, athletes are in recovery mode and preparing for the next training session or competition. It is clear that CHO repletion is of paramount importance, as most training sessions and competitions for endurance and stop-and-go sports require high muscle glycogen stores for fuel. The same can be said regarding the importance of ingesting protein after exercise in order to stimulate muscle protein synthesis and rapidly move the muscle into positive protein balance. There also has been growing evidence that recovery nutrition must consider the amount of fat that is consumed in order to replenish the IMTG stores that have been used during exercise. Trained athletes often have as much energy stored as IMTG as they do glycogen, and IMTGs are a significant source of fuel during prolonged low and moderate intensity exercise in untrained and trained men and women [10, 26]. Although it is unclear whether beginning an exercise session with a reduced IMTG store will limit the exercise capacity, an inability to replenish this store over repeated training sessions could lead to such a situation.

Several published studies have examined the time course of IMTG recovery following exercise that depleted a portion of the IMTG store. They demonstrate that recovery diets lasting 18–48 h that contain only 10–24% of the total energy intake as fat do not replenish IMTG as quickly as diets that contain higher fat intakes (35–57% of total energy). In fact, two studies reported no IMTG repletion after 18 h with repeated meals containing 21% fat [36] and 48 h where 24% fat was consumed [37]. On the other hand, the recovery of IMTG was complete after only 22 h when a 35% fat diet was consumed after exercise [37]. This study also reported that the exercise-induced decreases in IMTG content and the lack of IMTG replenishment in the low-fat trial was only in the type 1 fibers. It has been estimated that the amount of ingested fat required for IMTG repletion is ~2 g/kg body mass per day [38]. However, a high fat intake right after exercise may compromise the ability to replete muscle glycogen and impair performance, so a common strategy is to emphasize CHO and protein replenishment in the first 6–8 h after exercise, and then increase the fat content beyond this time point [38]. This may be a sound strategy as the replenishment of IMTG in the hours after exercise appears to be delayed by the fact that skeletal muscle oxidizes a large portion of the available FFA as the majority of ingested CHO is stored as glycogen. No changes in muscle IMTG levels were reported at 2, 3 or 6 h of recovery following exercise [36, 39, 40], while glycogen was substantially repleted [36].

Athletes who engage in prolonged exercise every day may have chronically low IMTG content, leaving them in a more CHO-dependent state where their post-exercise diet would require extra CHO. This may not matter as they prepare for an endurance event that requires exercise at a higher power output than training. In other words, is there ever a situation where a greater reliance on fat would benefit an endurance athlete's performance? Also, are there any benefits of training with higher or lower IMTG levels? These questions have not been answered and will be discussed in the following chapter.

Conclusions

The regulation of fat metabolism in skeletal muscle is complex and involves many sites of control. Recent work has identified the importance of fat transport across the plasma and mitochondrial membranes and the regulation of IMTG degradation as major sites of control regulating fat metabolism and oxidation during exercise. The oxidation of fat is maximal during moderate intensity exercise with distinct control mechanisms for downregulation of fat oxidation at intense aerobic intensities associated with high-level sports training and competitions. Exercise training is the most potent stimulus for increasing the muscle mitochondrial volume and the capacity to oxidize fat during exercise. Molecular work has identified that increases in transcriptional and mitochondrial proteins during training result from the cumulative effects of transient bursts in their mRNAs. Nutritional schemes that have attempted to acutely provide more FFA in the diet, increase adipose tissue lipolysis, and augment fat oxidation directly in the muscle have been largely unable to augment fat oxidation enough to substantially spare CHO use during exercise. In addition, the effects of these acute nutritional manipulations on the molecular responses in the muscle have been largely unexplored. Lastly, some work has investigated the importance of the fat content in recovery diets, but little is known about the consequences of these strategies for success in subsequent training sessions and competitions.

References

1 Asmussen E: Muscle metabolism during exercise in man. A historical survey; in Pernow B, Saltin B (eds): Muscle Metabolism during Exercise. New York, Plenum Press, 1971, pp 1–11.

2 Froberg SO, Mossfeldt F: Effect of prolonged strenuous exercise on the concentration of triglycerides, phospholipids, and glycogen in muscle of men. Acta Physiol Scand 1971;82:167–171.

3 Havel RJ, Pernow B, Jones NL: Uptake and release of free fatty acids and other metabolites in the legs of exercising men. J Appl Physiol 1967;23:90–99.

4 Hoppeler H, Luthi P, Claassen H, et al : The ultrastructure of the normal human skeletal muscle. A morphometric analysis on untrained men, women and well-trained orienteerers. Pflugers Arch 1973;344:217–232.

5 Romijn JA, Coyle EF, Sidossis LS, et al: Regulation of endogenous fat and carbohydrate metabolism in relation to exercise intensity and duration. Am J Physiol 1993;265:E380–E391.

6 VanLoon LJ, Greenhaff PL, Constantin-Teodosiu D, et al: The effects of increasing exercise intensity on muscle fuel utilization in humans. J Physiol 2001;536:295–304.

7 Zimmermann R, Strauss JG, Haemmerle G, et al: Fat mobilization in adipose tissue is promoted by adipose triglyceride lipase. Science 2004;306:1383–1386.

8 Nickerson, JG, Alkhateeb H, Benton CR, et al: Greater transport efficiencies of the membrane fatty acid transporters FAT/CD36 and FATP4 than FABPpm and FATP1, and differential effects on fatty acid esterification and oxidation in rat skeletal muscle. J Biol Chem 2009;201:199–209.

9 Glatz JF, Luiken JJ, Bonen A: Membrane fatty acid transporters as regulators of lipid metabolism: implications for metabolic disease. Physiol Rev 2010;90:367–417.

10 Stellingwerff T, Boon H, Jonkers RS, et al: Significant intramyocellular lipid use during prolonged cycling in endurance-trained males as assessed by three different methodologies. Am J Physiol 2007;292:E1715–E1723.

11 Watt MJ, Heigenhauser GJF, Spriet LL: Effects of dynamic exercise intensity on the activation of hormone-sensitive lipase in human skeletal muscle. J Physiol 2003;547:301–308.

12 Watt MJ, Heigenhauser GJF, Dyck DJ, Spriet LL: Intramuscular triacyglycerol, glycogen and acetyl group metabolism during 4 h of moderate exercise. J Physiol 2002;541:969–978.

13 Holloway GP, Bezaire V, Heigenhauser GJ, et al: Mitochondrial long chain fatty acid oxidation, fatty acid translocase/CD36 content and carnitine palmitoyltransferase I activity in human skeletal muscle during aerobic exercise. J Physiol 2006;571:201–210.

14 Stephens FB, Constantin-Teodosiu D, Greenhaff PL: New insights concerning the role of carnitine in the regulation of fuel metabolism in skeletal muscle. J Physiol 2007;581:431–444.

15 Romijn JA, Coyle EF, Sidossis LS, et al: Relationship between fatty acid delivery and fatty acid oxidation during strenuous exercise. J Appl Physiol 1995;79:1939–1945.

16 Starritt EC, Howlett RA, Heigenhauser GJF, et al: Sensitivity of CPT I activity to malonyl-CoA in trained and untrained human skeletal muscle. Am J Physiol 2000;278:E462–E468.

17 Holloszy JO: Biochemical adaptations in muscle. Effects of exercise on mitochondrial oxygen uptake and respiratory enzyme activity in skeletal muscle. J Biol Chem 1967;242:2278–2282.

18 Holloszy JO, Coyle EF: Adaptations of skeletal muscle to endurance exercise and their metabolic consequences. J Appl Physiol 1984;56:831–838.

19 Gollnick PD, Armstrong RB, Saubert CWT, et al: Enzyme activity and fiber composition in skeletal muscle of untrained and trained men. J Appl Physiol 1972;33:312–319.

20 Booth F, Neufer PD: Exercise genomics and proteomics; in Tipton CM (ed): ACSM's Advanced Exercise Physiology. Baltimore, Lippincott Williams & Wilkins, 2006, pp 623–651.

21 Schmitt B, Fluck M, Decombaz J, et al: Transcriptional adaptations of lipid metabolism in tibialis anterior muscle of endurance-trained athletes. Physiol Genomics 2003; 15:148–157.

22 Perry CGR, Lally J, Holloway GP, et al: The time-course of molecular responses associated with mitochondrial biogenesis during training in human skeletal muscle. J Physiol 2010;588:4795–4810.

23 Perry CGR, Heigenhauser GJF, Bonen A, et al: High-intensity aerobic interval training increases fat and carbohydrate metabolic capacities in human skeletal muscle. Appl Physiol Nutr Metab 2008;33:1112–1123.

24 Holloway GP, Spriet LL: Skeletal muscle metabolic adaptations to training; in: Maughan RJ (ed): The Olympic Textbook of Science in Sport. Oxford, Wiley-Blackwell, 2009, pp 70–83.

25 Talanian JL, Holloway GP, Snook L, et al: Exercise training increases sarcolemmal and mitochondrial fatty acid transport proteins in human skeletal muscle. Am J Physiol Endocrinol Metab 2010;299:E180–E188.

26 Schrauwen-Hinderling VB, Hesselink MKC, Schrauwen P, et al: Intramyocellular lipid content in human skeletal muscle. Obesity 2006;14:357–367.

27 Alsted TJ, Nybo L, Schweiger M, et al: Adipose triglyceride lipase in human skeletal muscle is upregulated by exercise training. Am J Physiol Endocrinol Metab 2009;296:E445–E453.

28 Gibala M: Molecular responses to high-intensity interval training. Appl Physiol Nutr Met 2009;34:428–432.

29 Dyck DJ, Putman CT, Heigenhauser GJ, et al: Regulation of fat-carbohydrate interaction in skeletal muscle during intense aerobic cycling. Am J Physiol 1993;265:E852–E859.

30 Chesley A, Howlett RA, Heigenhauser GJF: Regulation of muscle glycogenolytic flux during intense aerobic exercise following caffeine ingestion. Am J Physiol 1998;275:R596–R603.

31 Sidossis LS, Gastaldelli A, Klein S, et al: Regulation of plasma fatty acid oxidation during low- and high-intensity exercise. Am J Physiol 1997;272:E1065–E1070.

32 Massicotte D, Peronnet F, Brisson GR, et al: Oxidation of exogenous medium-chain free fatty acids during prolonged exercise: comparison with glucose. J Appl Physiol 1992;73:1334–1339.

33 Putman CT, Spriet LL, Hultman E, et al: Skeletal muscle pyruvate dehydrogenase activity during acetate infusion in humans. Am J Physiol 1995;268:E1007–E1017.

34 Jeukendrup AE, Saris WHM, Brouns FR, et al: Effects of carbohydrate (CHO) and fat supplementation on CHO metabolism during prolonged exercise. Met 1996;45:915–921.

35 Decombaz J, Arnoud MJ, Milon H, et al: Energy metabolism of medium chain triglycerides versus carbohydrate during exercise. Eur J Appl Physiol 1983;52:9–14.

36 Kimber NE, Heigenhauser GJF, Spriet LL,
    et al: Skeletal muscle fat and carbohydrate
    metabolism during recovery from glycogen
    depleting exercise in humans. J Physiol
    2003;548:919–928.
37 Van Loon LJC, Schrauwen-Hinderling VB,
    Koopman R, et al: Influence of prolonged
    endurance exercise and recovery diet on
    intramuscular triglyceride content in trained
    males. Am J Physiol 2003;285:E804–E811.
38 Decombaz J: Nutrition and recovery of
    muscle energy stores after exercise. Sportmed
    Sporttraumatol 2003;51:31–38.
39 VanLoon LJC, Koopman R, Stegen JHCH, et
    al: Intramyocellular lipids form an important
    substrate source during moderate intensity
    exercise in endurance-trained males in a
    fasted state. J Physiol 2003;553:611–623.
40 VanHall G, Sacchetti M, Redegran G, et al:
    Human skeletal muscle fatty acid and glyc-
    erol metabolism during rest, exercise and
    recovery. J Physiol 2002;543:1047–1058.

Discussion

Dr. Hoppeler: You say you can increase fat metabolism during exercise when the fat content in the blood stream is acutely increased (e.g. by using heparin). To me this suggests that the muscle plasma membrane is a very severe barrier or else the limitation to fat use is within the muscle fiber.

Dr. Spriet: The conclusion is actually the opposite – because simply increasing the free fatty acid concentration restores a good portion of the fat oxidation that was lost when going from 40 to 80% VO_{2max} (plasma FFA level is low at 80% VO_{2max}). The largest barrier to fat oxidation during intense exercise lies in the adipose tissue. However, it doesn't look like it is adipose lipolysis per se, because measurements of lipolysis suggest that it stays high at high exercise intensities. Instead, it appears that a reduction in blood flow within adipose tissue limits the amount of fat that gets out into the bloodstream and binds to albumin. However, fat oxidation doesn't get restored all the way back up to the levels seen at lower intensity exercise, suggesting that there are also some limitations either for fat coming into the muscle cell or for fat getting to the mitochondria. Most of the fat that comes into the muscle during exercise goes straight to the mitochondria for oxidation and is not cycled through IMTG. This points the finger at the adipose tissue as well as the muscle in terms of explaining the decreased fat oxidation when moving from a moderate to heavy exercise intensity.

Dr. Hoppeler: Some migratory birds completely rely on fat metabolism during migratory flights when they exercise at a very high intensity. Is it known how this amazing feat is achieved?

Dr. Spriet: McFarlan et al. [1] recently reported that birds have a very good ability to oxidize fat during migration and a very high concentration of fat transport proteins in skeletal muscle. From an evolutionary point of view, fat is a good fuel when you work at a high intensity against gravity as these birds do, because of the amount of energy per gram of stored substrate. They reported a large upregulation of muscle fat transport proteins in the migratory vs. non-migratory seasons. It seems that exercise training in humans does not induce similar changes, and humans are not capable of the high rates of fat oxidation at high exercise intensities that these animals achieve during migration. It would seem that the evolutionary pressure to successfully migrate has driven the changes to maximize fat oxidation.

Dr. Phillips: With respect to your zero change in IMTG content after exercise – you said that there was no net use, but you can't measure breakdown and synthesis with a static measure of content.

Dr. Spriet: Yes, that is correct. We cannot say whether fat coming into the muscle is first esterified to IMTG and whether some lipolysis is also occurring. However, there is no net change in content during the recovery period, meaning that the fat used is ultimately coming from outside the cell. There has been an argument that recovery requires a net use of IMTG, but we have not seen this [2].

Dr. Phillips: Pulse tracer methods as used by Jensen [3] provide data that seem to be fairly robust; why has nobody followed up on that in human beings?

Dr. Spriet: It has been done in humans, but it's hard to do, and there is some concern about how accurate the pulse chase tracer methodology is. It appears that the fat that is added to IMTG in the pulse phase is the first to break down during the chase phase, rather than fully equilibrating with all IMTG. This would lead to erroneously high values of FFA-IMTG cycling, but we cannot be sure whether or not that's actually the case. Data from Jensen's lab indicate that at rest there is a lot of simultaneous IMTG synthesis and breakdown.

Dr. Phillips: Indeed at 50% VO_{2max} they show inward and outward flux but no net change in the pool.

Dr. Spriet: Yes, and those results do not match findings from other laboratories where there is net use of IMTG in exercise at ~50% VO_{2max} that lasts more than 1 h. I suppose that there is some futile cycling, but in their first paper they suggested that 93% of the fat that came into the muscle cell from outside was immediately oxidized during exercise and only 7% was esterified to IMTG [3]. Why it would go through IMTG first and then be oxidized in an exercise situation remains unclear to me. This would make sense during rest as has been shown by a recent paper from their laboratory [4], but during exercise the incoming FFAs need to be oxidized.

Dr. Phillips: The tracer studies suggest that you need to activate lipoprotein lipase to make use of circulating triglycerides. The main regulation of lipoprotein lipases is through insulin, which is very low during exercise. This could be why it is not possible to get too much out of these.

Dr. Spriet: Epinephrine might play a role in some tissues, but it does not appear that this regulation is very powerful in skeletal muscle. We don't know all the regulators of plasma TG degradation, but it seems that skeletal muscle is not designed to make much use of circulating triglycerides, especially as we move to higher exercise intensities. At higher intensities, you don't even have to give an intralipid solution; heparin injections alone will cause an activation of LPL and raise the circulating FFA levels (50–60% of the response you get if you add additional TG from an intralipid infusion). The Scandinavian groups argue that the provision of FFA from circulating TGs does play a role, but of course they don't really measure it, and simply deduce it from their other measurements and assume what they cannot account for is circulating TGs.

Dr. Maughan: You wrote in your manuscript that muscle can function with no carbohydrate. Is it really true that all of the energy can come from fat?

Dr. Spriet: I can't answer that question, but if you do the classic experiment and deplete the muscle of carbohydrate as much as you can, and then put subjects on a high fat diet for two and half days, they have very little glycogen in their muscles. However, there is some carbohydrate and that's where that statement comes from. So, clearly there is a small amount of carbohydrate, but it's as minimal as you can possibly make it. In the experiment I described above, subjects begin exercise with muscle glycogen in the order of 100–200 mmol per kg dry muscle and they are lasting about 30–35 min during exercise at ~75% VO_{2max}. Although some carbohydrate is used at the beginning of exercise, there is little available in the later stages, and they have to rely on what they can get from outside the cell. Invariably, these people have no glycogen in their muscle and are hypoglycemic when they reach volitional exhaustion.

Dr. Maughan: You said, the most powerful stimuli to increase fat oxidation are aerobic training and high fat feeding, but what about fasting? Is the high fat feeding really more effective than fasting? Is it not the absence of carbohydrate that is increasing fat oxidation?

Dr. Spriet: Yes, you can add fasting too. I don't know who would do it in the real world, but I suppose there are athletes who may try this.

Dr. Maughan: But there is more than just a conceptual difference. Is it the fact that carbohydrate is not available that promotes fat use or is there something about fat feeding that promotes fat utilization by muscle?

Dr. Spriet: We can argue over whether removing carbohydrate is more important than providing extra fat, but it's virtually impossible to separate the two in an intact person. Taking away carbohydrate suppresses insulin, which is believed to be a signal to downregulate key enzymes in carbohydrate metabolism, like pyruvate dehydrogenase. High fat diets quickly increase free fatty acid levels, which enter the cell and activate transcriptional factors to increase proteins associated with fat metabolism. However, your point is well taken as the body is very sensitive to the lack of carbohydrate. When no carbohydrate has been ingested for a few hours, the activity of pyruvate dehydrogenase in all the tissues will decrease rapidly, and this probably occurs during overnight sleep.

Dr. Hawley: Bengt Saltin and John Holloszy say that one of the major factors driving mitochondrial biogenesis is the post-exercise elevation in free fatty acids. You showed very nicely in your study that FFAs are hugely elevated in this situation. Going back to the point of triggers for adaptation – should we withhold carbohydrate after exercise, because as soon as you ingest carbohydrate you decrease fat metabolism. Shouldn't we train intensely with glycogen on board and then proceed with starvation to maintain increased fat availability?

Dr. Spriet: With respect to prolonging the increases in the plasma FFAs after exercise, I don't have an answer to that. However, in the rat model that John Holloszy uses, he keeps the FFA levels high for a long period of time and can show mitochondrial biogenesis. However, when working with humans, it does not seem practical to keep the FFA concentration high for 4 h instead of the normal 1–1.5 h, for example.

Dr. Hawley: A paper has just come out in rats from Winder's lab [5], where exercise was mimicked by AICAR treatment, and rats were given high-fat diets. It was found that AMPK activation by AICAR and a high-fat diet had an additive effect in some muscle tissue.

Dr. Spriet: Yes, I am aware of the use of the so-called 'exercise mimetics' like AICAR. However, we have to keep in mind that the exercise stimulus is very powerful on its own. For example, in the study cited in my talk we used untrained people, and exercised them for 4 min at 90% VO_{2max}, followed by 2 min of rest, and repeated this procedure 10 times, with workouts every other day. This is indeed a very large stimulus. There is not much you can do to make a person train harder. It may help if you breathe a hyperoxic gas mixture under these training conditions, as it seems to have a central effect such that you can train at about 25 W greater during your entire training protocol – so 275 instead of 250 W in normoxia. Yet, all the muscle measurements we made at various time points during the training regimen looked identical, suggesting that the extra 25 W didn't add any additional training stimulus, presumably because the insult or training stimulus of the normal training was so great. This might be quite different if you try to further stimulate mitochondrial biogenesis in well-trained athletes; hyperoxia may be more favorable under these conditions.

Dr. Hawley: A comment regarding the excellent Perry et al. [6] paper. If you look at the PGC1-α mRNA responses over the 7 days of training, this response is dropping, suggesting that you need more overload to restore the training effect.

Dr. Spriet: Yes, you may be correct, but PGC1-β starts to increase after about 5 or 7 days, so PGC1-β might be playing a role later on in training. But you are correct, there could be a downregulation of the PGC1-α response over time, and the same exercise stimulus may not have the same effect as training progresses. This needs to be explored in training protocols.

Dr. van Loon: I would like to go back to the possibility that extracellular fat availability might limit fat oxidation during high-intensity exercise. Data published in the past showed that with high intensity exercise there is still an increase in free fatty acids in the cytosol. So, it doesn't seem to be anything extracellular that is limiting, and that goes hand to hand with the rest of your data. If you increase fat provision by intralipid infusion and see an increase in fat oxidation from 40 to 80% maximum work load capacity, that doesn't mean that the fat load is limiting fat oxidation. It just means that if you go from 40 to 60% you would see an increase in fat oxidation, whereas if you go from 60 to 80% you wouldn't see it. Many people have misinterpreted our previous study, looking at the contribution of the different endogenous fat sources during exercise of various exercise intensities [7]. Besides plasma free fatty acid oxidation, we quantified the use of 'other fat sources'. These other fat sources include everything that is not coming from the plasma and should therefore include both intramuscular triglycerides and plasma lipids. However, the use of plasma lipids is already largely represented by the use of plasma free fatty acids. Due to their high turnover, plasma lipids become rapidly enriched to the same level as the plasma free fatty acids. So, what you consider to be plasma free fatty acid oxidation also includes the use of plasma triglycerides.

Dr. Spriet: So, all the so-called 'other' sources should be labeled intramuscular? With respect to the importance of free fatty acids inside the cell, the reason I didn't mention these is that the contribution from these and the actual concentration within the cell is pretty controversial. I am not sure that I would hang my hat on that just yet.

Dr. van Loon: Following exercise, you see a continuous increase in free fatty acid levels, and the flux continues for 15 min after exercise and then drops. This suggests that plasma free fatty acid provision is quite in line with the amount that the muscle would like to access. So, lipid fuel supply seems to be better organized than what we generally think.

Dr. Spriet: Much of the confusion comes from the fact that we are looking for ways to get athletes who work at very high intensities to rely more on fat so they can spare carbohydrate for carbohydrate-dependent aspects later in the competition. However, unlike the migrating bird, the human body is simply not designed to rely heavily on fat oxidation at high exercise intensities.

Dr. van Loon: We see direct correlations between the amount of IMTG oxidation, oxidative capacity and performance, so many people, including ourselves, have tried to optimize IMTG storage. But IMTGs might simply be a representation of fluxes in fatty acids because if you reduce the free fatty acid flux you start oxidizing more IMTGs. IMTGs could thus be viewed as a reserve storage depot when the plasma provision of lipids is insufficient to allow maximal fat oxidation rates.

Dr. Spriet: Exactly, and that's what we have seen as well. During 4 h of exercise at 55% VO_{2max}, most IMTG is used in the first hour. As soon as the athlete can mobilize free fatty acids to fairly high levels, plasma FFAs become the dominant fat source and the reliance on IMTGs decreases.

Dr. van Loon: So, IMTG are an important substrate source but not to allow maximal oxidation.

Dr. Spriet: Yes, but if you look at some of the data following 8 h of submaximal exercise, the IMTG concentrations are essentially used up. So, over this prolonged exercise you continue to use some IMTG.

Dr. Hoppeler: We showed long ago that running 100 km results in an almost complete loss of IMTGs [8].

Dr. Baar: I was going to say the same thing, especially in the birds because what you see in the birds is a huge increase in intramuscular triglyceride as they prepare to migrate, to a point where you actually see a disruption of the myofibrillar lattice to some degree. I think it's because it's just a readily available source.

Dr. Maughan: How is the story on the regulation of substrate metabolism in cardiac muscle, is it very different from skeletal muscle?

Dr. Spriet: I don't know, as I have not followed the cardiac literature very closely. Obviously the heart relies more heavily on exogenous free fatty acids. There are some big differences between the heart and skeletal muscle in terms of the way it's regulated, but I haven't been following that topic.

Dr. van Loon: IMTG levels in heart are high in obesity and in type 2 diabetes, but in athletes they are actually quite low. So, while athletes have high IMTG stores in skeletal muscles, they don't seem to have those in the heart.

Dr. Spriet: That fits fairly well with the whole body being under siege in people that are overweight. They simply have too much fat to dispose of, and it simply goes everywhere it can possibly go – in the liver, in the heart, in skeletal muscle, and in adipose tissue.

Dr. Gibala: Is the migration of the fat transport protein, FAT/CD36 in the plasma membrane exercise intensity dependent?

Dr. Spriet: We don't know that yet. We should repeat some of the studies that we have published and have people exercise at 40, 65 and then 90% of VO_{2max}. Especially if you begin exercise at 65% and then have athletes work at 85% for 30 min or whatever they can handle to see whether CD36 would just sit in the membrane or whether it would actually move back out of the membrane as the reliance on fat decreases. We also don't know anything about the time course of fat transport proteins moving out of the membranes after exercise, which could be interesting.

Dr. van Loon: Could you also discuss the experiments in which carnitine content of the muscle was increased?

Dr. Spriet: Recent work from Greenhaff's laboratory suggests that increasing muscle carnitine increases fat oxidation during exercise. However, there are a couple of problems with those studies. Firstly, insulin infusion is needed along with high levels of plasma carnitine to get additional carnitine into the muscle. Of course, high insulin levels cause many other metabolic changes – one is that it moves more FAT/CD36 to the muscle and mitochondrial membranes. This sets up the alternate hypothesis that it's not increasing carnitine that augments fat oxidation, but an increase in the transport of free fatty acid into the cell or into the mitochondria to be oxidized. This could be tested of course. Secondly, other evidence speaks against carnitine being limiting for fat oxidation: carnitine is not consumed in the process of moving fat into the mitochondria, and the highest levels of fat oxidation (~65% VO_{2max}) occur when muscle carnitine levels are already quite low. In addition, if the plasma free fatty acid concentration is artificially raised to high levels during intense exercise, the muscle oxidizes more fat, again suggesting that carnitine is not limiting. However, as with many metabolic processes, all these factors could work together to downregulate fat utilization at high workloads. It makes a lot of sense from a teleological point of view to shift to carbohydrate as a fuel when exercise intensity is close to the limit of your oxygen uptake ability, to get as much energy as possible from each liter of oxygen consumed.

References

1 McFarlan JT, Bonen A, Guglielmo CG: Seasonal upregulation of fatty acid transporters in flight muscles of migratory white-throated sparrows (Zonotrichia albicollis). J Exp Biol 2009;212:2934–2940.

2 Kimber NE, Heigenhauser GJF, Spriet LL, et al: Skeletal muscle fat and carbohydrate metabolism during recovery from glycogen depleting exercise in humans. J Physiol 2003;548:919–928.

3 Guo Z, Burguera B, Jensen MD: Kinetics of intramuscular triglyceride fatty acids in exercising humans. J Appl Physiol 2000;89:2057–2064.

4 Kanaley JA, Shadid S, Sheehan MT, et al: Relationship between plasma free fatty acid, intramyocellular triglycerides and long-chain acylcarnitines in resting humans. J Physiol 2009;587:5939–5950.

5 Fillmore N, Jacobs DL, Mills DB, et al: Chronic AMP-activated protein kinase activation and a high-fat diet have an additive effect on mitochondria in rat skeletal muscle. J Appl Physiol 2010;109:511–520.

6 Perry CGR, Lally J, Holloway GP, et al: The time-course of molecular responses associated with mitochondrial biogenesis during training in human skeletal muscle. J Physiol 2010;588:4795–4810.

7 VanLoon LJ, Greenhaff PL, Constantin-Teodosiu D, et al: The effects of increasing exercise intensity on muscle fuel utilization in humans. J Physiol 2001;536:295–304.

8 Oberholzer F, Claassen H, Moesch H, et al: Ultrastructural, biochemical and energy analysis of extreme duration performance (100 km run). Schweiz Z Sportmed 1976;24:71–98.

Maughan RJ, Burke LM (eds): Sports Nutrition: More Than Just Calories – Triggers for Adaptation.
Nestlé Nutr Inst Workshop Ser, vol 69, pp 59–77,
Nestec Ltd., Vevey/S. Karger AG., Basel, © 2011

Fat Adaptation Science: Low-Carbohydrate, High-Fat Diets to Alter Fuel Utilization and Promote Training Adaptation

John A. Hawley

Health Innovations Research Institute, School of Medical Sciences, RMIT University,
Bundoora, VIC, Australia

Abstract

The effect of manipulating an individual's habitual diet on skeletal muscle fuel utilization
has been of longstanding interest to scientists, and it is now well established that changes
in dietary intake that alter the concentration of blood-borne substrates and hormones
cause substantial perturbations in the macronutrient storage profile of muscle and exert
profound effects on rates of substrate oxidation during exercise. Only recently, however,
has it become appreciated that nutrient-exercise interventions can modulate many
contraction-induced responses in muscle, and that fuel availability per se provides a 'trigger' for adaptation. Consumption of low-carbohydrate, high-fat diets in the face of endurance training alters patterns of fuel utilization and subsequent exercise responses. Human
studies show how low-carbohydrate, fat-rich diets interact with specific contractile stimulus to modulate many of the acute responses to exercise, thereby promoting or inhibiting
subsequent training adaptation.   Copyright © 2011 Nestec Ltd., Vevey/S. Karger AG, Basel

Introduction

The impact of manipulating an individual's habitual diet on skeletal muscle fuel
utilization during exercise has been of longstanding interest to scientists. Classic
studies conducted at the turn of the 20th century provided the first compre-
hensive information on the interactive effects of diet and contractile activity on
muscle metabolism. The main findings from these investigations were that: (1)
both fat- and carbohydrate (CHO)-based fuels were oxidized by the working

muscles during submaximal exercise, with the contribution from fat decreasing as exercise intensity increased; (2) changes in an individual's preceding diet altered resting muscle metabolism and patterns of fuel oxidation during subsequent exercise, and (3) humans have a low capacity for exercise when fat-based fuels are the major energy source. In the 1930s, researchers in Scandinavia provided further evidence of diet-exercise interactions, specifically how training status and exercise duration affected patterns of fuel utilization during strenuous physical activity. The findings from these pioneering studies underpin our current understanding of muscle fuel metabolism during exercise [1].

It is now well established that changes in dietary intake that alter the concentration of blood-borne substrates and hormones cause large perturbations in the macronutrient storage profile of skeletal muscle (and other insulin-sensitive tissues) and exert profound effects on fuel use during exercise. Only recently, however, has it been appreciated that nutrient-exercise interventions can modulate many contraction-induced responses in muscle [2–4] and that fuel availability per se provides a 'trigger' for adaptation. This chapter provides a contemporary perspective on how consumption of a low-CHO, high-fat diet combined with strenuous physical activity alters patterns of fuel utilization and subsequent exercise responses. Emphasis will be on the results of human studies and how fat-rich diets interact with specific contractile stimulus to modulate many of the acute responses to exercise, thereby promoting or inhibiting subsequent training adaptation.

Effects of High-Fat Diets on Fuel Utilization during Exercise

The effect of consuming a high-fat (60–65% of energy intake, 4–5 g/kg body mass per day), low-CHO (<20% of energy intake, 2 g/kg body mass per day) diet for less than 3 days is to lower resting muscle and liver glycogen concentrations and increase rates of whole-body fat oxidation during moderate intensity (60–75% of maximal O_2 uptake, VO_{2max}) exercise. It should be noted, though, that muscle glycogen levels are well preserved even during fasting in the absence of exercise. Such short-term exposure to a low-CHO, fat-rich diet is detrimental to training capacity and endurance performance [5, 6], presumably due to a combination of lowered muscle glycogen stores in the absence of any worthwhile increase in the capacity of the muscle to oxidize fat to compensate for the reduction in endogenous CHO availability. However, consumption of high-fat, low-CHO diets for longer periods (i.e. 1–7 weeks) elicits metabolic adaptations that significantly enhance rates of fat oxidation during both low and intense (>85% of VO_{2max}) exercise and, to a large extent, compensate for the diet-induced reduction in CHO availability.

In one of the longest exposures to a fat-rich diet, Helge et al. [7] studied 13 untrained male subjects who performed 7 weeks of endurance training (3–4 sessions per week) while consuming either a high-fat (n = 7) or a high-CHO diet (n = 6). Before and after the training-diet intervention, subjects performed 60 min of submaximal cycling during which stable isotopes (1-^{13}C palmitate), combined with whole-body gas exchange and muscle and blood measures were employed to determine substrate kinetics. RER values were lower in subjects who had consumed the high fat diet than those consuming the high-CHO diet (0.86 vs. 0.93 units; $p < 0.05$), with the majority of this increased fat oxidation being derived from a higher uptake of plasma fatty acids (FAs) by muscle and also a large uptake of very low-density lipoprotein triacylglycerol. The decreased CHO oxidation (so-called 'carbohydrate sparing') during the 60-min exercise bout was entirely due to a reduction in the rate of muscle glycogenolysis (2.6 ± 0.5 vs. 4.8 ± 0.5 mmol/kg dry mass per minute, $p < 0.05$) and not to a diminished plasma glucose uptake. However, it should be noted that the high-fat diet reduced resting (i.e. pre-exercise) muscle glycogen levels compared to the high-CHO diet (480 ± 29 vs. 683 ± 46 mmol/kg dry mass, $p < 0.05$). Glycogen 'sparing' can only be substantiated if subjects commence standardized exercise with similar muscle glycogen stores after both high-fat and high-CHO diets [5].

Effects of a High-Fat Diet and Carbohydrate Restoration on Fuel Utilization during Exercise

In 1995, Hawley and Hopkins [8] proposed that 'optimal endurance and ultra-endurance performance may be attained if an athlete trains for most of the year on a high-CHO diet, then, one week before a major event, undergoes a short (5-day) period of fat adaptation, followed by 24–36 h of a high-CHO intake to restore muscle and liver glycogen stores.' Such 'dietary periodization' could, in theory, allow athletes to maximize endogenous fuel stores (muscle glycogen and triacylglycerol, and liver glycogen), optimize the contribution from both aerobic lipolytic and glycolytic pathways to oxidative metabolism, and 'spare' muscle glycogen [8]. To test this hypothesis, we have undertaken a series of independent but related studies using a standardized dietary-exercise intervention protocol (a 5- to 6-day period of either a high-fat or isoenergetic high-CHO diet consumed while subjects undertake strenuous training followed by 24 h of rest and high CHO intake) in association with prolonged, steady-state cycling (to allow for measures of substrate oxidation) and training and performance responses [9–15].

Figure 1 summarizes metabolic data from Burke et al. [9], and shows RER values along with rates of whole-body CHO and fat oxidation measured during 20 min of submaximal cycling at baseline (day 1), after 5 days of fat adaptation (day 6), and finally during 120 min of steady-state exercise after one day of rest and a high-CHO diet (day 7) or 6 days of an energy-matched high-CHO diet.

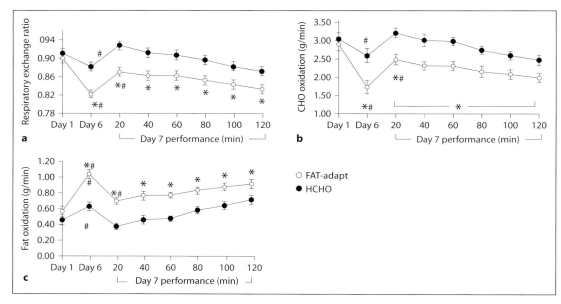

Fig. 1. The effect of 5 days of consumption of a high-fat diet and one day of CHO restoration (Fat-adapt) on respiratory exchange ratio (**a**), whole-body rates of CHO oxidation (**b**), and fat oxidation (**c**) during 20 min of continuous cycling at 70% of maximal oxygen uptake, compared with 6 days of a high-CHO diet (HCHO). Values are means ± SE for 8 well-trained male subjects on day 1 (baseline), on day 6 (adaptation), and during 120 min of continuous steady-state cycling on day 7. Comparison of data for 20 min of cycling (day 1 vs. day 6 vs. day 7): [#] $p < 0.05$, different from day 1; * $p < 0.05$, different from HCHO. Comparison of data from 120 min of steady-state cycling during performance ride: * $p < 0.05$, different from HCHO. Data are from Burke et al. [9]. Reproduced with the permission of the American Physiological Society.

Five days of strenuous training while consuming either diet reduced RER values, so that on day 6 values were lower than on day one. However, the RER after fat adaptation was lower than with the high-CHO diet (0.82 ± 0.01 vs. 0.88 ± 0.01; $p < 0.05$). Muscle glycogen levels after 5 days of a high-fat diet were significantly lower than on day 1 (255 ± 24 vs. 451 ± 32 mmol/kg dry weight; $p < 0.05$) and also lower than after 5 days on a high-CHO diet (464 ± 42 mmol/ kg dry weight; $p < 0.05$). One day of high-CHO diet and rest increased muscle glycogen values for both dietary treatments (to 554 ± 45 and 608 ± 51 mmol/kg dry mass for fat adaptation and high CHO, respectively). This 'carbohydrate restoration' was associated with an increase in RER values for both treatments, but RER values were still lower than values on day 1 after fat adaptation (0.87 ± 0.01 vs. 0.90 ± 0.01; $p < 0.05$) and below the corresponding values for the high-CHO diet (0.93 ± 0.01, $p < 0.05$). Although there was a progressive decline in RER values during the 120 min of exercise undertaken on day 7 with both treatments,

RER values after fat adaptation remained lower than during the high-CHO trial at all corresponding time points [9].

Five days of low-CHO, high-fat intake increased rates of fat oxidation during submaximal exercise (fig. 1). On day 6 of fat adaptation, rates of fat oxidation were almost twofold higher than values observed on day 1 (1.04 ± 0.07 vs. 0.57 ± 0.07 g/min; $p < 0.05$) and were greater than the corresponding values for the high-CHO trial (0.63 ± 0.06 g/min; $p < 0.05$). Although one day of rest and high-CHO intake attenuated the rates of fat oxidation during the first 20 min of exercise on day 7, fat oxidation remained elevated above baseline (day 1; $p < 0.05$) and above rates measured in the high-CHO trial (0.70 ± 0.05 vs. 0.37 ± 0.04 g/min; $p < 0.05$). Fat oxidation increased over 120 min of cycling with both treatments, but was higher after fat adaptation at all time points [9].

It is interesting to observe that despite the brevity of the adaptation period (5 days), a low-CHO, energy-sufficient diet induces substantially higher rates of FA oxidation (compared to baseline) in trained athletes who already have a high capacity for fat oxidation and may have been expected to have maximized training-induced adaptations for FA metabolism. Of note was that a subsequent investigation revealed that elevated rates of fat oxidation persist even under conditions in which CHO availability was increased by either having athletes consume a high-CHO meal before commencing exercise [10] and/or ingesting glucose solutions during exercise [10, 13]. Thus, 5 days of a high-fat diet consumed in the face of vigorous training induces powerful metabolic adaptations within skeletal muscle that upregulate FA oxidation independent of both endogenous and exogenous CHO availability. Using a combination of serial muscle biopsies and glucose tracer methodology, we were able to show that the reduction in CHO oxidation during submaximal exercise was almost entirely accounted for by a true 'sparing' of muscle glycogen stores: both total blood glucose oxidation and rates of ingested glucose oxidation were similar during exercise after both high-fat and high-CHO interventions [9, 10, 15].

The investigations of the effects of low-CHO, high-fat diets from our lab [9–15] have all utilized competitive athletes who continue to train intensely while consuming diets containing a higher proportion of fat (4 g/kg per day, 65% of energy) than they would habitually ingest. Vogt et al. [16] determined whether some of the metabolic adaptations that result from such extreme diets can be obtained if athletes ingest diets in which the fat content is within the range typically chosen by trained individuals. These workers [16] studied 11 duathletes who ingested a low-CHO, high-fat (50–55% of energy) diet for 5 weeks while undertaking their normal training regimen. Resting muscle glycogen content was not different between the two diets (488 ± 38 vs. 534 ± 33 mmol/kg dry weight for high-fat and high-CHO diet, respectively), but the high-fat diet resulted in a twofold increase in resting muscle triacyglcerol content. Blood lactate concentrations and RER values were lower after the low-CHO, high-fat diet at rest and during a range of submaximal exercise tests. However, in accordance with previous findings [9, 10, 12], a variety of performance tests were not different after either diet intervention [16].

What Mechanisms Explain the Increased Rates of Fat Oxidation after High-Fat Diets?

Several metabolic adaptations in skeletal muscle contribute to the increased rates of whole-body fat oxidation and decreased rates of CHO oxidation observed after fat adaptation strategies. With regard to FA metabolism, fat-rich diets facilitate an increase in rates of whole-body lipolysis and an increased FA response at rest and during exercise [16], in part due to higher circulating catecholamine concentrations [7]. The elevated FA levels at rest and during exercise, in association with lower muscle glycogen stores are likely to underlie the elevated muscle triacyglycerol content seen after fat adaptation [7, 15, 16]. Elevated circulating FA levels are also likely to drive increased enzymatic activities such as greater concentrations of β-hydroxyacyl-CoA-dehydrogenase, carnitine palmitoyl-transferase I (CPT I) and hormone-sensitive lipase [14, 17, 18] as well as modulating the expression of mRNA-encoding proteins necessary for FA transport, such as FA translocase [11].

As would be expected, there were reciprocal changes in CHO metabolism, with high-fat diets reducing resting muscle glycogen concentration [10, 15] and presumably liver glycogen stores to some degree. As noted earlier, the reduction in CHO oxidation observed after fat adaptation and CHO restoration is due to a sparing of muscle glycogen [10, 15]. While such 'sparing' should, in theory, be beneficial for endurance exercise capacity, fat adaptation strategies have not been demonstrated to provide a clear benefit to the performance of prolonged exercise [5, 6]. One reason to explain this paradox is that fat adaptation protocols directly inhibit rates of muscle glycogenolysis during exercise. In this regard, Stellingwerff et al. [14] reported that 5 days of a high-fat diet followed by one day of 'carbohydrate restoration' suppressed resting levels of pyruvate dehydrogenase (PDHa) activity by ~60% compared to an isoenergetic high-CHO diet for 6 days (0.39 ± 0.10 vs. 0.82 ± 0.18 mmol/kg wet weight per minute). In response to a bout of submaximal cycling undertaken on day 7 (20 min at 70% of VO_{2max}), there was a rapid increase in PDHa activity which, although similar after both diet interventions, remained 29% lower at the end of exercise after fat adaptation (1.69 ± 0.25 vs. 2.39 ± 0.19 mmol/kg wet weight per minute; $p = 0.003$). Even in a 60-second sprint, an exercise challenge that would be expected to maximally activate muscle glycogenolysis, PDHa activity remained suppressed after fat adaptation ($p < 0.05$), even though the relative increase in PDH activation during the 1-min sprint was similar between dietary treatments (~35%). As a result of less pyruvate oxidation (via a reduced PDH flux), estimates of glycogenolysis during both the first minute of submaximal exercise and the supramaximal sprint were also lower after fat adaptation [14]. While the precise metabolic signals responsible for the shift in muscle substrate use during submaximal and supra-maximal cycling after fat adaptation are not known, it is clear that they are likely to involve both an upregulation of processes involved in FA metabolism, as well as downregulation of CHO oxidation pathways.

Interaction of Training and High-Fat Diets on Training Adaptation

Helge et al. [19] were the first to study the interaction of training and a high-fat diet on metabolism and training capacity. These workers studied 20 young, healthy males who ingested either a high-fat (n = 10) or a high-CHO (n = 10) diet while performing endurance training 3–4 times a week for 7 weeks. During the 8th week, both groups ingested a high-CHO diet. Endurance performance conducted at the completion of the 7th week of the training program revealed a significantly greater improvement after a CHO-rich diet has been consumed during training compared to a fat-rich diet (56%). Even when the high-fat diet was replaced by a high-CHO diet for the 8th week of training, endurance performance was still significantly lower than in subjects who had trained for the complete duration on a high-CHO diet. They [19] concluded that 'ingesting a fat-rich diet during an endurance training programme is detrimental to endurance performance (. . .) due to suboptimal adaptations that are not remedied by the short-term increase in carbohydrate availability.'

From a practical perspective, it seems unlikely that fat oxidation can match the energy demands of the strenuous training undertaken by competitive endurance and ultra-endurance athletes. To test this hypothesis, Stepto et al. [13] determined the effect of consuming a high-fat diet for 4 days on the training responses of competitive ultra-endurance cyclists/triathletes with a history of prolonged endurance training. These subjects were either national or international level athletes, with 3 of them completing the Hawaii Ironman World Championships within weeks of study completion. During the 4-day intervention period, subjects performed two high-intensity cycle interval training sessions in the laboratory (consisting of a 20-min warm up at 65% of VO_{2max} followed by 8 × 5 min work bouts at 85% of VO_{2max} with 60 s recovery at 100 W), during which pulmonary gas exchange measures were taken at regular intervals to allow for estimates of fuel oxidation. The other two training sessions consisted of 2- to 4-hour easy rides on the road (fig. 2).

Rates of fat oxidation during the 20-min warm up (undertaken at a power output of 232 W) were 69 ± 25 μmol/kg per minute [14]. These values are in close agreement with the 57 μmol/kg per minute we have previously reported for competitive endurance athletes cycling at 70% of VO_{2max} (234 W) after 5 days of a fat-rich diet [10]. However, despite an increase in both the relative and absolute exercise intensity when undertaking the intense interval workout

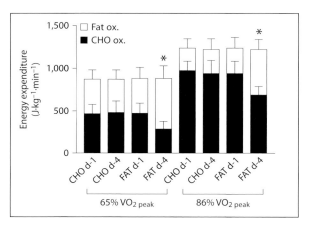

Fig. 2. Energy expenditure estimated from pulmonary gas measurements during 20 min of cycling at 65% of maximal oxygen uptake [VO_{2max}] and during a high-intensity interval training session (performed at 86% of VO_{2max}, 323 ± 32 W) for day 1 and day 4 of either a high-fat (FAT) or high-CHO (CHO) diet. * $p < 0.05$, different to CHO d-1, and FAT, d-1,. Data are from Stepto et al. [13]. Reproduced with the permission of Lippincott, Williams and Wilkins.

(ridden at an average power output of 323 ± 32 W), rates of fat oxidation did not decline [14]. This indicates that after 4 days of a high-fat diet, well-trained athletes were better able to oxidize fat during high-intensity exercise to compensate for their low muscle glycogen stores. Although subjects in that study [14] were able to complete the prescribed training regimen while consuming a high-fat diet, this was associated with a significant increase in perceived effort for both laboratory and on-road sessions. This suggests that consumption of a fat-rich diet for a longer intervention period would limit the ability of well-trained athletes to undertake strenuous training.

Does Training with Increased Fat Availability Augment Skeletal Muscle Adaptation?

Endurance training is associated with an increase in the activities of key enzymes of the mitochondrial electron transport chain and a concomitant increase in mitochondrial protein content. These biochemical and morphological changes, along with an increased capillary supply and blood flow, result in a shift in trained muscle to a greater reliance on fat as a fuel with a concomitant reduction in glycolytic flux and tighter control of acid-base status. High-fat diets and interventions that chronically elevate plasma FA concentrations (i.e. heparin injections) induce adaptations in skeletal muscle that mimic endurance training (e.g. activate transcription of genes encoding enzymes involved in FA oxidation and increase the capacity of muscle to oxidize FA). The mechanisms by which exercise and increased FA availability activate mitochondrial biogenesis appear to be distinct [20], but it has been proposed that the 5′ adenosine monophosphate-activated protein kinase (AMPK) may provide a link between training- and nutrient-induced adaptations in skeletal muscle [21]. Evidence for such a premise comes from the results of both human and animal studies in which AMPK activity has been shown to be modulated by both contraction (i.e. exercise) and substrate availability (i.e. muscle glycogen and triacylglycerol stores and circulating FA levels).

AMPK is a member of a metabolite-sensing protein kinase family that exists as a heterotrimer formed by three subunits α, β and γ. The α catalytic and β regulatory subunits exist in two isoforms ($α_1$, $α_2$, $β_1$, $β_2$) while the γ subunit exists in three ($γ_1$, $γ_2$ and $γ_3$). This structure allows for twelve possible combinations of the AMPK complex due to the fact that each subunit is encoded by multiple genes subjected to alternative splicing [20]. AMPK functions as a metabolic 'fuel gauge' in skeletal muscle; activation in response to decreased energy levels (i.e. muscle contraction) inhibits ATP-consuming pathways and activates pathways involved in CHO and FA catabolism to restore ATP levels. AMPK promotes FA oxidation in skeletal muscle during exercise by inhibiting acetyl-CoA carboxylase (ACC-β) and activating malonyl-CoA, thus removing inhibition of mitochondrial fatty acyl-CoA translocation by CPT I. Numerous studies have reported that these exercise-induced effects on ACC-β and malonyl-CoA are closely paralleled by activation of AMPK.

AMPK induces mitochondrial biogenesis by increasing the ability of the peroxisome proliferator-activated receptor-γ coactivator (PGC-1α) to coactivate transcription factors that regulate the coordinated expression of mitochondrial proteins encoded in the nuclear and mitochondrial genomes. Indeed, AMPK directly phosphorylates and activates PGC-1α. Overexpression of PGC-1α in muscle results in a large increase in functional mitochondria, while a single bout of exercise induces a rapid increase in PGC-1α in skeletal muscle [22]. In contrast, high-fat feeding and/or increased circulating FAs are thought to promote mitochondrial gene transcription by regulating PGC-1α via different mechanisms. Raising circulating FAs increase the peroxisome proliferator-activated receptor co-activators (PPARs) which regulate expression of the mitochondrial FA oxidative enzymes [23] and lead to a posttranscriptional increase in PGC-1α protein [24]. Specifically, PPARα induces an increase in the expression of proteins involved in transport and metabolism of FA [25], while activation or overexpression of the PPARδ has been reported to result in an increase in mitochondrial biogenesis in muscle [26].

A single bout of prolonged exercise is associated with an increase in both AMPK activity and elevations in circulating FAs; so, an important question is whether chronic exercise undertaken with elevated FA availability has an additive effect on skeletal muscle training adaptation (i.e. mitochondrial biogenesis). We recently reported an increase in AMPK-α_2 but not -α_1 activity in rodent skeletal muscle in response to chronic high-fat feeding [27]. In that study, AMPK-α_1 activity was only increased when animals concurrently undertook an intense endurance training program while consuming a high-fat diet [27]. At the time, we suggested distinct roles for the AMPK-α subunit in skeletal muscle, with AMPK-α_1 activity being linked to exercise training-induced adaptations and CHO availability (i.e. muscle glycogen storage), and AMPK-α_2 activity being responsive to increased lipid availability (i.e. muscle triacyglycerol stores and circulating FAs). Further evidence in support of this hypothesis comes from the results of Yeo et al. [15]. These workers reported a strong relationship between resting AMPK-α_2 activity (but not -α_1) and muscle triglyceride content in humans consuming a fat-rich diet and undertaking strenuous training. In contrast, AMPK-α_1 (but not -α_2) was associated with increased muscle glycogen content in that study [15].

Recently, Fillmore et al. [20] determined if chronic AMPK activation in skeletal muscle (via a chemical activator of AMPK, 5-aminoimidazole-4-carboxamide riboside [AICAR]), and high-fat diet-induced elevations in blood FAs had an additive effect on mitochondrial content of skeletal muscle. Rats were treated for 6 weeks with AICAR injections, a high-fat diet, or both AICAR injections and a high-fat diet. They reported additive effects of AICAR and high-fat feeding on markers of FA metabolism, the citric acid cycle, the electron transport chain, and transcriptional regulation. However, these changes were confined to muscles with low oxidative capacity [20]. Such an observation is of note, because prolonged endurance training in humans is typically associated with a reliance on slow-twitch muscle fibers with a high oxidative capacity. This suggests that there are species-specific differences with regard to the interactive effects of training and high-fat diets. Indeed, the majority of human studies that have examined the interaction of training and a high-fat diet fail to demonstrate a beneficial effect on either enzymatic responses and/or endurance capacity [10, 12, 18, 19]. Part of the difference in results between rodent and human studies may be due to differences in habitual macronutrient intake of fat: the typical Western diet consists of ~35–40% fat, and it is possible that further elevations in dietary lipid intake would be less likely to enhance mitochondrial biogenesis than if the fat content of the regular diet was closer to the typical 'control' diets consumed by rats [20]. Alternatively, few human studies examine fiber type-specific responses to diet-training interventions, and when sampling mixed muscle (usually the vastus lateralis), any potential differential effects are likely to have been overlooked.

As noted previously, other signaling proteins regulate expression of the mitochondrial FA oxidative enzymes in response to changes in circulating FAs. In humans, Horowitz et al. [28] reported an increased PPARα skeletal muscle protein expression in 5 untrained middle aged women after ~3 months of endurance training, while Russell et al. [29] found that PPARα protein was higher in 7 healthy males after 6 weeks of endurance training. Both of these studies were undertaken while subjects consumed moderate- to high-CHO diets. In contrast, Helge et al. [30] studied 13 men who trained one leg for 4 weeks (~30 h of total exercise), while the other leg remained untrained. During the intervention period, 6 subjects consumed a high-fat diet (58% of energy intake as fat, 24% CHO), while the remainder maintained their normal diet (33% fat, 56% CHO). Muscle biopsies were obtained from vastus lateralis in both legs before and after training. Despite a lower RER during standardized submaximal exercise in both untrained and trained legs in subjects who consumed the high-fat diet, PPARα mRNA abundance and protein expression remained unchanged [30]. They [30] concluded that 'a longer and more intense training programme may be required to induce changes in PPARα expression'. However, we reported that in rat muscle, PPARα and PPARγ protein expression is unaltered after 8 weeks exposure to a high-fat diet [31]. Taken collectively, the results from these studies suggest that the PPARs may play only a permissive role in modulating training adaptation in the face of increased fat availability.

Conclusions

The consumption of a fat-rich diet for less than 3 days is associated with reduced muscle glycogen stores in subjects who continue to train and increased rates of FA oxidation during low- to moderate-intensity exercise. Such short-term fat diets are detrimental to endurance capacity and the performance of prolonged exercise. In contrast, longer (1–7 weeks) periods of high-fat intake in combination with regular endurance training elicit metabolic adaptations in muscle that markedly increase rates of fat oxidation during both low- and high-intensity exercise and, to a large extent, compensate for the diet-induced reduction in CHO availability. Yet, despite marked changes in metabolism that favor fat oxidation and 'spare' muscle glycogen oxidation, fat adaptation strategies do not provide clear benefits to training capacity or endurance performance. The mechanisms by which exercise and increased FA availability activate mitochondrial biogenesis appear to be different, but likely involve the AMP kinase and possibly the PPARs. While fat adaptation, CHO restoration protocols offer scientists a unique human model to investigate the interactive effects of alterations in fuel availability on muscle metabolism during exercise, high-fat diets are associated with the development of muscle insulin resistance, a condition that is not compensated for by the diet-induced increases in fat oxidation and/ or mitochondrial biogenesis. Accordingly, caution should be exercised when recommending high-fat diets to athletes.

Acknowledgements

Studies of fat adaptation undertaken in the author's laboratory have been funded by grants from the Australian Sports Commission and Nestlé Australia. The author would like to thank Drs. Trent Stellingwerff, Lawrence Spriet and Ronald Maughan for constructive comments in the preparation of the manuscript.

References

1 Kiens B, Hawley J: Fat metabolism; in Stear S, Shirreffs S (ed): Nutrition Society Textbook on Sport & Exercise Nutrition. Oxford, Wiley-Blackwell, 2011.

2 Hawley JA, Burke LM: Carbohydrate availability and training adaptation: effects on cell metabolism and exercise capacity. Exerc Sport Sci Rev 2010;38:152–160.

3 Hawley JA, Burke LM, Phillips SM, Spriet LL: Nutritional modulation of training-induced skeletal muscle adaptation. J Appl Physiol 2011;110:834–845.

4 Hawley JA, Tipton KD, Millard-Stafford ML: Promoting training adaptations through nutritional interventions. J Sports Sci 2006; 24:709–721.

5 Burke LM, Hawley JA: Effects of short-term fat adaptation on metabolism and performance of prolonged exercise. Med Sci Sports Exerc 2002;34:1492–1498.

6 Helge JW: Adaptation to a fat-rich diet: effects on endurance performance in humans. Sports Med 2000;30:347–357.

7 Helge JW, Watt PW, Richter EA, et al: Fat utilization during exercise: adaptation to a fat-rich diet increases utilization of plasma fatty acids and very low density lipoprotein-triacylglycerol in humans. J Physiol 2001;537: 1009–1020.

8 Hawley JA, Hopkins WG: Aerobic glycolytic and aerobic lipolytic power systems. A new paradigm with implications for endurance and ultraendurance events. Sports Med 1995; 19:240–250.

9 Burke LM, Angus DJ, Cox GR, et al: Effect of fat adaptation and carbohydrate restoration on metabolism and performance during prolonged cycling. J Appl Physiol 2000;89: 2413–2421.

10 Burke LM, Hawley JA, Angus DJ, et al: Adaptations to short-term high-fat diet persist during exercise despite high carbohydrate availability. Med Sci Sports Exerc 2002; 34:83–91.

11 Cameron-Smith D, Burke LM, Angus DJ, et al: A short-term, high-fat diet up-regulates lipid metabolism and gene expression in human skeletal muscle. Am J Clin Nutr 2003; 77:313–318.

12 Carey AL, Staudacher HM, Cummings NK, et al: Effects of fat adaptation and carbohydrate restoration on prolonged endurance exercise. J Appl Physiol 2001;91:115–122.

13 Stepto NK, Carey AL, Staudacher HM, et al: Effect of short-term fat adaptation on high-intensity training. Med Sci Sports Exerc 2002;34:449–455.

14 Stellingwerff T, Spriet LL, Watt MJ, et al: Decreased PDH activation and glycogenolysis during exercise following fat adaptation with carbohydrate restoration. Am J Physiol Endocrinol Metab 2006;290:E380–E388.

15 Yeo WK, Lessard SJ, Chen ZP, et al: Fat adaptation followed by carbohydrate restoration increases AMPK activity in skeletal muscle from trained humans. J Appl Physiol 2008; 105:1519–1526.

16 Vogt M, Puntschart A, Howald H, et al: Effects of dietary fat on muscle substrates, metabolism, and performance in athletes. Med Sci Sports Exerc 2003;35:952–960.

17 Phinnney SD, Bistrian BR, Evans WJ, et al: The human metabolic response to chronic ketosis without caloric restriction: preservation of submaximal exercise capacity with reduced carbohydrate oxidation. Metabolism 1983;32:769–776.

18 Helge JW, Kiens B: Muscle enzyme activity in humans: role of substrate availability and training. Am J Physiol 1997;41: R1620–R1624.

19 Helge JW, Richter EA, Kiens B: Interaction of training and diet on metabolism and endurance during exercise in man. J Physiol 1996; 492:293–306.

20 Fillmore N, Jacobs DL, Mills DB, et al: Chronic AMP-activated protein kinase activation and a high-fat diet have an additive effect on mitochondria in rat skeletal muscle. J Appl Physiol 2010;109:511–520.

21 Hardie DG, Sakamoto K: AMPK: a key sensor of fuel and energy status in skeletal muscle. Physiology (Bethesda) 2006;21: 48–60.

22 Lin J, Handschin C, Spiegelman BM: Metabolic control through the PGC-1 family of transcription coactivators. Cell Metab 2005;1:361–370.

23 Kelly DP, Scarpulla RC: Transcriptional regulatory circuits controlling mitochondrial biogenesis and function. Genes Dev 2004; 18:357–368.

24 Hancock CR, Han D-H, Chen M, et al: High fat diets cause insulin resistance despite an increase in muscle mitochondria. Proc Natl Acad Sci U S A 2008;105:7815–7820.

25 Muoio DM, Way JM, Tanner CJ, et al: Peroxisome proliferator-activated receptor-alpha regulates fatty acid utilization in primary human skeletal muscle cells. Diabetes 2002;51:901–909.

26 Wang Y-X, Zhang C-L, Yu RT, et al: Regulation of muscle fiber type and running endurance by PPARδ. PLoS Biol 2004; 2:1532–1539.

27 Lessard SJ, Rivas DA, Chen ZP, et al: Tissue-specific effects of rosiglitazone and exercise in the treatment of lipid-induced insulin resistance. Diabetes 2007;56:1856–1864.

28 Horowitz JF, Leone TC, Feng W, et al: Effect of endurance training on lipid metabolism in women: a potential role for PPARalpha in the metabolic response to training. Am J Physiol Endocrinol Metab 2000;279:E348–E355.

29 Russell AP, Feilchenfeldt J, Schreiber S, et al: Endurance training in humans leads to fiber type-specific increases in levels of peroxisome proliferator-activated receptor-gamma coactivator-1 and peroxisome proliferator-activated receptor-alpha in skeletal muscle. Diabetes 2003;52:2874–2881.

30 Helge JW, Bentley D, Schjerling P, et al: Four weeks one-leg training and high fat diet does not alter PPARα protein or mRNA expression in human skeletal muscle. Eur J Appl Physiol 2007;101:105–114.

31 McAinch AJ, Lee JS, Bruce CR, et al: Dietary regulation of fat oxidative gene expression in different skeletal muscle fiber types. Obes Res 2003;11:1471–1479.

Discussion

Dr. Maughan: It's perhaps worth thinking hard about whether we are really talking about high-fat diets or whether the most important aspect of these diets is that they are low in carbohydrate. Supposing you fed your volunteers a diet with a normal (for them) amount of carbohydrate and supplemented the diet with fat so you had normal carbohydrate plus high fat, would you see the same effect?

Dr. Hawley: It's important to know whether these are trained or untrained subjects, because the absolute capacity for fat oxidation differs greatly. It probably also depends on the subjects' training load. Training sessions that deplete muscle glycogen may give a very different response from studies where subjects do just 30 min a day of light- to moderate-intensity aerobic exercise. Exercise with low muscle glycogen stores will increase the absolute and relative contribution from lipid-based fuels to oxidative metabolism. So to answer your question, I believe you would see an increase in fat metabolism when a 'normal' carbohydrate diet is supplemented with fat, at least in trained individuals. A study from Dr. Hoppeler's lab shows just this effect [1].

Dr. Maughan: But can we look at your studies in more detail? The papers by Stepto et al. [2] and Burke et al. [3], for example. Were the diets fed in these studies high-fat diets or low-carbohydrate diets?

Dr. Hawley: They were both! In these two investigations, the diets were low in carbohydrate (2.5 g/kg body mass per day) and high in fat (4 g/kg body mass per day). We gave that amount of carbohydrate because it was sufficient to maintain glycemia, yet resulted in low muscle glycogen levels at the onset of the intervention.

Dr. Maughan: But that is a low-carbohydrate diet. If you gave a normal diet with added fat – the same amount of fat – would training still be impaired? I am asking you to speculate as to the mechanism that is driving these effects. Feeding a low-carbohydrate diet has far greater metabolic and hormonal effects than feeding a high-fat diet.

Dr. Hawley: You are correct in that carbohydrate restriction is likely to have a more pronounced effect on the hormonal milieu than a high-fat diet. There is more than one candidate for the mechanism driving the training adaptation, but muscle glycogen concentration is a major factor determining transcription of some regulatory genes. As we discussed in a recent review [4], commencing selected training sessions when muscle glycogen concentration is low results in greater transcriptional activation of several genes with key roles in the adaptation process compared to undertaking the same exercise bout when muscle glycogen concentration is normal or high. As noted by Hansen et al. [5], this is probably because several transcription factors include glycogen-binding domains: when muscle glycogen is low, these factors are released and become free to associate with different targeting proteins. However, in some of the studies we recently reviewed [4], low-glycogen was not the only variable to be manipulated. For example, in several investigations, subjects trained twice daily on the low-glycogen treatment compared to daily when glycogen was normal: it may be that training frequency or indeed the recovery between workouts is also an important factor driving adaptation.

Dr. Phillips: What if you just took away some of the carbohydrate and replaced it with protein, or what if you just cut back total energy intake so that the subjects weren't getting sufficient carbohydrate from the standpoint of full repletion. Then you wouldn't have to manipulate fat.

Dr. Hawley: That's something we haven't considered. Of course, if you change energy intake, there is a whole new set of issues concerning the ability to train anyway! When carbohydrate intake is very low (e.g. 2–3 g/kg body mass per day), intense training sessions just go out the window. In the study by Stepto et al. [2], it was clear that unless we had used highly trained, highly motivated subjects, they would have quit the training sessions we prescribed fairly early on: they were having trouble sustaining any intensity over 70–75% of VO_{2max} after just 4 days of a low-carbohydrate, high-fat diet; so, it's my feeling that it would be impossible to go any longer than that.

Dr. Phillips: But let's go back to the original two times a day training model that created this whole high fat paradigm. It would seem that some of the adaptations taking place in muscle are quite beneficial for somebody who is overweight or who has metabolic syndrome or type 2 diabetes.

Dr. Hawley: Let's clarify something here. The original study by Hansen et al. [5] was actually entitled 'Skeletal muscle adaptation: training twice every second day vs. training once daily'. If you read that paper, they proposed the paradigm that some training sessions should be commenced with low muscle glycogen stores, not necessarily high fat availability (at least in their minds). And clearly, they thought that twice-a-day training was superior for promoting adaptation than once-a-day training. If you get motivated people with insulin resistance and/or type 2 diabetes to exercise twice a day three times a week rather than once a day five times a week (for the same total exercise time), you may well see a greater adaptation. I don't know if anyone has looked at the effects of this experimental model in obese individuals or in people with insulin resistant metabolic syndrome. Those are logical studies to do.

Dr. Maughan: But the trouble with changing the protein content of the diet is it's not the same experimental model because you shift acid-base status.

Dr. Phillips: That would depend in part on the protein that you used. Whey is very neutral, it's low in sulphur-containing amino acids, so you don't get much sulphuric acid production, and therefore you don't do a lot to pH.

Dr. Zemel: Can we clarify the nature of these high-fat diets? Just as when we are talking about protein, we talk about the nature of the protein and its amino acid composition, so when we raise the notion of high-fat diet, we should think about the nature of these fats. We have already addressed the issue of medium chain fatty acids, but there are several other issues related to the composition of fat. For example, α-linolenic acid is oxidized differently, or I should say preferentially, compared to other fatty acids.

Dr. Hawley: Prof. Louise Burke was responsible for the formulation of the diets in the human studies we did, so perhaps she can address your question. However, in a recent study in rats we fed diets containing fatty acids with different chain lengths [6]. As someone alluded to earlier in this meeting, changing the fatty acid composition of the diet changes the membrane phospholipids and many other aspects of cell metabolism. That is well known. We didn't measure acid-base parameters after the different diets, but these would probably change too.

Dr. Burke: We did think about changing the fatty acid composition of the diet. Work from Dr. Peters' lab [7] has examined this very question. They showed that elevated n-3 fatty acids in a high-fat diet attenuate the increase in PDH kinase activity but not PDH activity in human skeletal muscle. So, clearly changing the fatty acid composition of the diet has metabolic consequences. One thing that stopped us from taking this further was just the practicality of constructing diets that would give 250 g of fat while also providing an obligatory amount of carbohydrate. This is just unworkable; so, when we found that there was impairment of the training intensity and the capacity to train, we just gave up the battle. The information is interesting in the metabolic sense, but does not seem to change sports performance, so we moved on.

Dr. Hawley: That might be interesting in a clinical setting. These subjects have a tremendous capacity to oxidize fat. And these high-fat diets do not induce insulin resistance. We have done that study [8], and the insulin sensitivity of well-trained subjects consuming our high-fat diets doesn't change at all, at least in the short-term. As Dr. Burke noted, the modified diet that we used gave the metabolic effects that we were interested in, so we just kept the same diet for subsequent investigations.

Dr. Montain: Historically, there was always the concept that when you are on a high-fat diet you feel sluggish and don't want to move. What has been your observation of your subject population – did they experience the same sort of symptoms?

Dr. Hawley: Certainly, they felt sluggish and they didn't want to move: we had to encourage them to complete the training regimen. The training was very hard, and they wouldn't have done it voluntarily. The ratings of perceived exertion are high, although perhaps not as high as you might expect, and the high-intensity training is just agony. There is only a small amount of carbohydrate available at the onset of the interval training sessions and when you are doing these intense efforts (8 times 5-min work bouts at 85% of VO_{2max}) we know from previous studies that they deplete approximately 50% of muscle glycogen stores when you start with values around 400–500 mmol/kg dry mass [9]. So when you start the same session with muscle glycogen values of around 200 mmol/kg dry weight, you are obviously going to be in trouble.

Dr. Burke: In one of those studies, we blinded the diets. We were able to produce foods that looked identical and that tasted very similar, but by day 3, all of the subjects just felt so terrible with the low-carbohydrate high-fat diet that there was nothing we could do to disguise it.

Dr. Hawley: I had forgotten that study with the so-called 'decoy foods'. We gave them lots of strawberries and lots of lettuce: subjects perceived this as a healthy diet and associated it with carbohydrate but at the end of the intervention, they weren't fooled.

Dr. Hoppeler: What is really high-fat diet? We used an intervention on highly-trained subjects where we just changed the diet composition by going down to 20% fat, or up to 50% fat still changed RER values by about 20% [1]. Substrate metabolism changes significantly, but you can't maintain the glycogen levels. It is also clear that people are very different in their reaction to these diets. When you report the mean values, it seems that nobody improves on a high-fat diet, but when you look at the individuals, it's completely different. These observations are usually not reported because it is not at all clear what is happening in these individuals, but our bias is that people who like high-fat diets work better on those and vice versa.

Dr. Hawley: I tried to bring that point out in the paper, and you will have noted that we always plot the individual subjects' data in our papers. We do know from subjects who took part in more than one study that if you are a 'responder' then you are always a 'responder' in subsequent studies. In animal models for high-fat diets, where some of the enzymatic changes are much more profound than in humans, the extreme diets used are probably the main factor. In the human studies, the diet manipulations are not as extreme as in the animal models. You have shown that [1].

Dr. Hoppeler: Rats, dogs and also mice produce mitochondria when you feed them diets that are high in fat. This is well known. Humans just don't respond in the same way.

Dr. Hawley: The work from John Holloszy's lab clearly shows that increasing fatty acid availability induces mitochondrial biogenesis in rodent skeletal muscle [10]. However, I want to stress that mitochondrial biogenesis and insulin sensitivity don't go hand in hand. Again, work from Holloszy's lab clearly shows that high-fat diets cause insulin resistance despite an increase in mitochondrial biogenesis [11]. I think this whole issue about mitochondrial deficiency causing insulin resistance and type 2 diabetes is nonsense [12]. Although the response of humans to a high-fat diet is not as robust as rodents when it comes to induction of mitochondrial biogenesis, it's not totally absent.

Dr. Hoppeler: When we changed the fat content of the diet by going up to only 50% lipid, there was absolutely no mitochondrial biogenesis, but still they got the higher fat oxidation: they lowered RQ by 20 at 75% of VO_{2max}, so I think it really depends on what you call a high fat diet and it may be different when you don't go to the extreme.

Dr. Hawley: But again, I would still like to make the point quite clearly that you can induce mitochondrial biogenesis and still remain insulin resistant. There are five or six papers I can quote to support this.

Dr. Maughan: One of the differences may be that laboratory animals are typically fed a very constant diet at baseline, but human volunteers are different. The composition of the volunteers' normal diet at entry to the study can vary quite considerably in terms of the fat, protein and carbohydrate content. If you then put them all on a fixed experimental diet, this will be a much bigger change for some than for others. You said there were some people who responded differently from others. Was that related to the degree of change from their habitual diet?

Dr. Hawley: We looked at the subjects' habitual diet but couldn't see any relationship to whether they were 'responders' or not. The freely selected diets of these well-trained athletes were quite homogenous, and were high in carbohydrate (about 6 g/kg body mass per day). So, clearly their habitual diet does not predict the response. We couldn't see anything in the food questionnaires that would predict yes or no. We thought about looking at the response to a single high-fat meal: would one high-fat meal turn on different genes in different individuals and then predict adaptation? So we have got that in store but it may not show much. I would like to think it would.

Dr. Baar: What about the possibility of changing the timing of fat intake, rather than a drastic change in composition? If you gave a bolus of the right fat just at the end of an endurance exercise bout, it could then be used during the period of high fat uptake and oxidation. This might drive the adaptive response in the same way that we can do with leucine or protein meals following resistance exercise.

Dr. Hawley: It's a great idea. I don't know of any experimental evidence, but if you look at the discussion in the recent paper from Will Winder's lab [13], they think that the postexercise elevation in free fatty acids is an important factor driving training adaptation. I am sure it plays a part but, as discussed in my paper, it's probably not enough to drive all the things that we see.

Dr. Baar: It may depend on what markers you use for mitochondrial biogenesis. Do you use a specific marker for mitochondria or are you looking at fat oxidation enzymes that are within the mitochondria but might vary independently of total mitochondrial protein? It could be that when some investigators say there is no mitochondrial biogenesis and others say that there is, they are looking at different things. Another consideration is whether the proteins have different half-lives and therefore might change at different rates. All of these factors make it difficult to address what really is happening.

Dr. Hoppeler: When I say mitochondria, I mean mitochondrial volume actually measured with electron microscopy techniques, which is sort of a global protein assay for a functional entity. Within that, you can obviously change the protein composition so that you can modify substrate selection independent of the volume.

Dr. Baar: We think of mitochondrial biogenesis as an increase in mitochondrial DNA (mtDNA). For us, that's the gold standard even though the protein level is important. There should be some proportionality between the amount of mitochondrial protein and the DNA number. You want to have something that's relevant, and so we tend to measure mtDNA number, but we also measure a couple of protein markers: we look at fat oxidation enzymes independently to get an idea of whether these enzymes all shift in the same direction, or one is shifting to a greater extent.

Dr. Hawley: In our recent paper on low carbohydrate, high fat availability [14], we measured mtDNA by real-time PCR. mtDNA is a marker of mitochondrial volume and increases with training. In contrast to the increases in mitochondrial enzyme activities, we saw after training twice a day on the low-carbohydrate, high-fat regimen [14], mtDNA content and PGC-1α protein content were unchanged after both diet-training interventions. Of course, the small (approximately 15–20%) increases in maximum enzyme activity observed after training twice every second day could coincide with a small increase in mitochondrial volume that is not detectable through mtDNA analysis.

Dr. Baar: But you still saw the adaptation with fat oxidation, which means that it doesn't take more mitochondria to get more fat oxidation enzymes into those mitochondria.

Dr. Hawley: And as Dr. Spriet has pointed out, measuring maximum enzyme activity (such as β-hydroxy-acyl-CoA) is probably not the way to go. We need to look at the rate-limiting enzyme in the transfer of long-chain fatty acids into the mitochondria, CPT I. As we have recently noted [15], most previous studies have been limited to total muscle measures that provide no information regarding the compartment or location where the protein changes occurred. This is important for subsequent work in this area.

Dr. Maughan: There was a whole series of studies done in the early 1900s in the preparations that were going on for Polar expeditions. Nansen used sled dogs, so he did studies feeding the dogs and the men different diets because high-fat foods are much easier to carry than high carbohydrate foods. My recollection of these studies is that he found the dogs could perform well on a diet that was pretty much 100% fat (with a bit of protein) for many weeks, but the men could not walk for more than 12 h a day unless the diet contained some carbohydrate. Mike Stroud and Ranulph Fiennes recently tried to walk across the Antarctic, but they took a higher fat content to save weight and had some problems in the later stages. When we talk about endurance, maybe we should remember those very long endurance activities, with up to 12 h of fairly hard exercise per day. Possibly you can cope with a high fat in events like that if you have muscles that are well adapted to fat oxidation.

Dr. Baar: So, notwithstanding the interest of this type of model for helping to understand the mechanisms that underpin adaptation in the muscle, do you see any point in pursuing this for any type of benefit?

Dr. Hawley: Yes, if you are one of those people who respond positively, I do definitely. However, from the perspective of an athlete or coach, the picture is less certain. It doesn't enhance performance and you feel worse during training. The athlete and coach will close the door when they hear that. It's a useful model to look at some of the factors around cell and metabolic regulation.

Dr. Burke: We have to remember the conditions of that experiment, though. The subjects were fasted, and no carbohydrate intake was allowed during the exercise. This is not what happens in the real world, at least with the conventional sports that we work with. It may be different for some of the adventure ultra-endurance events.

Dr. Hawley: Again, as Dr. Maughan has pointed out, if you looked at a different 'performance' measure such as submaximal exercise time to exhaustion, you may get different results to those obtained after more intense (shorter duration) lab performance measures. If we had looked at exercise time to exhaustion in our studies, I am pretty sure that fat adaptation would have prolonged it. So, perhaps with different exercise models, we might have reached different conclusions.

References

1 Vogt M, Puntschart A, Howald H, et al: Effects of dietary fat on muscle substrates, metabolism, and performance in athletes. Med Sci Sports Exerc 2003;35:952–960.

2 Stepto NK, Carey AL, Staudacher HM, et al: Effect of short-term fat adaptation on high-intensity training. Med Sci Sports Exerc 2002;34:449–455.

3 Burke LM, Angus DJ, Cox GR, et al: Effect of fat adaptation and carbohydrate restoration on metabolism and performance during prolonged cycling. J Appl Physiol 2000;89:2413–2421.

4 Hawley JA, Burke LM: Carbohydrate availability and training adaptation: effects on cell metabolism and exercise capacity. Exerc Sport Sci Rev 2010;38:152–160.

5 Hansen AK, Fischer CP, et al: Skeletal muscle adaptation: training twice every second day vs. training once daily. J Appl Physiol 2005;98:93–99.

6 Mitchell TW, Turner N, Else PL, et al: The effect of exercise on the skeletal muscle phospholipidome of rats fed a high-fat diet. Int J Mol Sci 2010;11:3954–3964.

7 Turvey EA, Heigenhauser GJ, Parolin M, Peters SJ: Elevated n-3 fatty acids in a high-fat diet attenuate the increase in PDH kinase activity but not PDH activity in human skeletal muscle. J Appl Physiol 2005;98:350–355.

8 Staudacher HM, Carey AL, Cummings NK, et al: Short-term high-fat diet alters substrate utilization during exercise but not glucose tolerance in highly trained athletes. Int J Sport Nutr Exerc Metab 2001;11:273–286.

9 Stepto NK, Martin DT, Fallon KE, Hawley JA: Metabolic demands of intense aerobic interval training in competitive cyclists. Med Sci Sports Exerc 2001;33:303–310.

10 Garcia-Roves P, Huss JM, Han DH: Raising plasma fatty acid concentration induces increased biogenesis of mitochondria in skeletal muscle. Proc Natl Acad Sci U S A 2007;104:10709–10713.

11 Hancock CR, Han D-H, Chen M, et al: High fat diets cause insulin resistance despite an increase in muscle mitochondria. Proc Natl Acad Sci U S A 2008;105:7815–7820.

12 Holloszy JO: Skeletal muscle "mitochondrial deficiency" does not mediate insulin resistance. Am J Clin Nutr 2009;89:463S–466S.

13 Fillmore N, Jacobs DL, Mills DB, et al: Chronic AMP-activated protein kinase activation and a high-fat diet have an additive effect on mitochondria in rat skeletal muscle. J Appl Physiol 2010;109:511–520.

14 Yeo WK, Paton CD, Garnham AP, et al: Skeletal muscle adaptation and performance responses to once a day versus twice every second day endurance training regimens. J Appl Physiol 2008;105:1462–1470.

15 Yeo WK, Carey AL, Burke L, et al: Fat adaptation in well-trained athletes: effects on cell metabolism. Appl Physiol Nutr Metab 2011;36:12–22.

Protein

Maughan RJ, Burke LM (eds): Sports Nutrition: More Than Just Calories – Triggers for Adaptation.
Nestlé Nutr Inst Workshop Ser, vol 69, pp 79–95,
Nestec Ltd., Vevey/S. Karger AG., Basel, © 2011

Dietary Protein to Support Muscle Hypertrophy

Luc J.C. van Loon[a] · Martin J. Gibala[b]

[a]Department of Human Movement Sciences, NUTRIM School for Nutrition, Toxicology and Metabolism, Maastricht University Medical Centre+, Maastricht, The Netherlands; [b]Exercise Metabolism Research Group, Department of Kinesiology, McMaster University, Hamilton, ON, Canada

Abstract

Intact protein, protein hydrolysates, and free amino acids are popular ingredients in contemporary sports nutrition, and have been suggested to augment post-exercise recovery. Protein and/or amino acid ingestion stimulates skeletal muscle protein synthesis, inhibits protein breakdown and, as such, stimulates muscle protein accretion following resistance and endurance type exercise. This has been suggested to lead to a greater adaptive response to each successive exercise bout, resulting in more effective muscle reconditioning. Despite limited evidence, some basic guidelines can be defined regarding the preferred type, amount, and timing of dietary protein that should be ingested to maximize post-exercise muscle protein accretion. Whey protein seems most effective in stimulating muscle protein synthesis during acute post-exercise recovery. This is likely attributable to its rapid digestion and absorption kinetics and specific amino acid composition. Ingestion of approximately 20 g protein during and/or immediately after exercise is sufficient to maximize post-exercise muscle protein synthesis rates. Coingestion of a large amount of carbohydrate or free leucine is not warranted to further augment post-exercise muscle protein synthesis when ample protein is already ingested. Future research should focus on the relevance of the acute anabolic response following exercise to optimize the skeletal muscle adaptive response to exercise training.

Introduction

Next to a certain genetic predisposition and regular participation in a well-designed training regimen, nutrition plays a key factor in determining physical well-being and exercise performance capacity. Good nutritional practice becomes even more important as athletes approach their limits with respect to training volume and intensity. This has renewed the interest among athletes, coaches, and exercise physiologists in the role of nutrition and nutritional modulation on physical performance. Specific nutritional interventions, including the use of specifically designed sports nutrition products, are widely used by athletes in an effort to compensate for the metabolic demands imposed upon by intense exercise training and/or competition. To improve endurance exercise performance capacity, dietary interventions generally aim to maximize endogenous carbohydrate availability before, during and/or after exercise. For this purpose, numerous carbohydrate-based sports drinks, energy bars and gels have been developed. In contrast, to enhance performance capacity in resistance type exercise tasks, nutritional interventions generally focus on stimulating muscle protein synthesis and/or reducing protein breakdown to augment the skeletal muscle adaptive response. This brief review will discuss the impact of dietary protein administration during acute post-exercise recovery and its proposed impact on the muscle adaptive response to exercise training. Consequently, this review will define some basic guidelines regarding the preferred type, amount, and timing of dietary protein administration to maximize post-exercise muscle protein accretion. Finally, limitations of the presented research and suggestions for future research to more successfully apply dietary protein administration to improve skeletal muscle reconditioning during exercise training will be discussed.

Post-Exercise Muscle Protein Synthesis and Breakdown

For muscle hypertrophy to occur, muscle protein synthesis rates must exceed muscle protein breakdown rates over a given period of time. Resistance exercise training is an effective interventional strategy to stimulate muscle protein synthesis. A single bout of resistance type exercise has been reported to stimulate skeletal muscle protein synthesis for up to 24–48 h [1, 2]. Resistance type exercise also stimulates muscle protein breakdown rates, albeit to a lesser extent than protein synthesis, and thus resistance type exercise effectively improves muscle protein balance. However, net protein balance remains negative in the absence of nutrient intake. The ingestion of carbohydrate and protein during post-exercise recovery further augments muscle protein synthesis and inhibits protein breakdown, resulting in net muscle protein accretion. Nutrition therefore forms a key factor in determining the effect of exercise training on muscle hypertrophy.

Carbohydrate ingestion during post-exercise recovery is an effective intervention to inhibit exercise-stimulated muscle protein breakdown, but does not seem to affect muscle protein synthesis [3, 4]. Though post-exercise protein

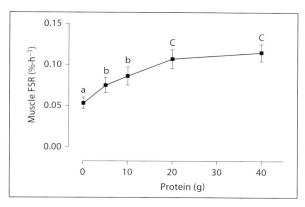

Fig. 1. Dose-response relationship between the amount of protein ingested and post-exercise muscle protein synthesis rates. Values represent means ± SEM. Means with different letters are significantly different from each other. FSR = Fractional synthesis rate. Figure reproduced from Moore et al. [20].

balance will improve following the ingestion of carbohydrate, net protein balance will remain negative [3]. The inhibitory effect of carbohydrate ingestion on post-exercise muscle protein breakdown has largely been attributed to the concomitant rise in circulating plasma insulin concentrations. However, even though elevated plasma insulin levels have been reported to stimulate net muscle protein anabolism, these properties are evident only in the presence of increased amino acid availability [5]. Recent studies support the contention that insulin is not a major regulatory factor determining muscle protein balance and identify amino acid availability as being the main stimulus for muscle protein synthesis under normal, resting conditions [6].

It has been established that protein/amino acid administration effectively stimulates muscle protein synthesis. Biolo et al. [7] demonstrated that hyperaminoacidemia, following intravenous amino acid infusion, increased post-exercise muscle protein synthesis rate and suppressed the exercise-induced increase in protein breakdown. Thereafter, Tipton et al. [8] showed that post-exercise ingestion of 40 g of either mixed amino acids (MAA) or essential amino acids only (EAA) also effectively stimulated muscle protein synthesis. Follow-up studies assessed the impact of smaller amounts of EAA with and without carbohydrate and showed that these were also effective in stimulating post-exercise muscle protein synthesis, resulting in a positive net protein balance during acute post-exercise recovery [9, 10]. Numerous other studies have shown that amino acid and/or protein administration increases muscle protein synthesis rates following resistance type exercise [3, 9–16]. Furthermore, amino acid and/or protein administration has also been shown to increase mixed muscle protein synthesis rates following endurance type exercise [17–19].

Amount of Dietary Protein

Though it has been well established that protein ingestion effectively stimulates muscle protein synthesis rates both at rest and following exercise, there is still considerable debate regarding the exact amount and type of protein and the desired timing of protein ingestion to maximize post-exercise muscle protein synthesis. Tipton et al. [8] showed that post-exercise ingestion of 40 g MAA or EAA effectively stimulated muscle protein synthesis. Since the ingestion of 40 g MAA or 40 g EAA resulted in a similar net protein balance, it was suggested that it might not be necessary to ingest nonessential amino acids during immediate post-exercise recovery. Follow-up studies assessed the impact of only 6 g EAA with and without carbohydrate and showed that this amount was also effective in stimulating post-exercise muscle protein synthesis. However, ingestion of such a small amount of EAA after exercise resulted in a positive net protein balance for up to 2 h only, after which net protein balance became negative again [9]. This suggests that ingestion of such an amount of amino acids is not sufficient to remain in an anabolic state. Recently, Moore et al. [20] conducted a dose-response study to investigate the relationship between protein ingestion and post-exercise muscle protein synthesis. The fractional synthetic rate of mixed muscle protein increased with the ingestion of greater amounts of protein, reaching maximal stimulation after 20 g intact (egg) protein, which provided approximately 8.6 g EAA. The authors speculated that athletes should ingest this amount of dietary protein 5–6 times daily to maximize skeletal muscle protein accretion on a habitual basis.

Source of Dietary Protein

Various studies have reported improved post-exercise protein balance and/or greater muscle protein synthesis rates following the ingestion of whey protein [21], casein protein [21], soy protein [22], casein protein hydrolysate [12, 23], egg protein [20], and whole-milk and/or fat-free milk [22, 24]. It seems obvious to question which source of dietary protein would be most effective to promote post-exercise muscle protein anabolism. While research comparing the efficacy of different proteins on the post-exercise protein synthetic response is slowly emerging, it is presently not possible to identify a specific protein source that is most effective for promoting post-exercise muscle protein accretion. The issue is further complicated by the fact that numerous parameters modulate the muscle protein synthetic response to protein ingestion during post-exercise recovery. The type, intensity, and duration of exercise prior to protein ingestion, the duration of the recovery period that is being assessed, the amount and timing of protein administration, the amino acid composition of the protein, and the digestion and absorption kinetics of the protein source (or mixed meal) provided, may all modulate the postprandial muscle protein anabolic response. To date, few studies have tried to assess differences in the post-exercise protein anabolic response to the ingestion of different types of protein.

Milk protein and its main isolated constituents, whey and casein, seem to offer an anabolic advantage over soy protein for promoting muscle hypertrophy [22, 25, 26]. Casein and whey protein seem to have distinct anabolic properties, which are attributed to differences in digestion and absorption kinetics [21, 27–29]. Whereas whey protein is a soluble protein that leads to fast intestinal absorption, intact casein clots in the stomach delaying its digestion and absorption and the subsequent release of amino acids in the circulation [30]. The fast, but transient rise in plasma amino acid concentration after whey protein ingestion can lead to higher protein synthesis and oxidation rates [21, 27–29]. Despite these differences, Tipton et al. [21] found no difference in net protein balance during recovery from resistance type exercise following casein versus whey consumption. In addition to intrinsic differences in digestion and absorption rate, it has been suggested that whey protein can more effectively stimulate protein synthesis due to its greater leucine content when compared to casein [25]. However, the latter may be questioned as Koopman et al. [12, 23, 31] showed that coingestion of free leucine did not further increase muscle protein synthesis rate when an ample amount of casein hydrolysate is ingested during post-exercise recovery. Additional studies are warranted to assess the impact of the digestion and absorption kinetics of a protein source and its amino acid composition on stimulating muscle protein synthesis rates following exercise. In accordance, the influence of the timing of protein administration should be considered when defining nutritional strategies to augment post-exercise muscle protein accretion.

Carbohydrate Coingestion

Post-exercise nutritional interventions should aim to enhance recovery and facilitate the adaptive response to regular exercise training. In the endurance trained athlete, rapid restoration of depleted muscle glycogen stores is generally a priority to enhance post-exercise recovery and thereby maintain performance capacity. Therefore, endurance trained athletes mainly focus on carbohydrate ingestion for post-exercise recovery. Recently, coingestion of relative small amounts of protein and/or amino acids has become popular among these athletes, mainly because this can further accelerate muscle glycogen repletion when less than optimum amounts of carbohydrate (<1.0 g/kg bodyweight per hour) are ingested.

As protein and/or amino acid ingestion has been proven essential to allow net muscle protein accretion following exercise [3, 12, 13, 23], athletes involved in resistance type exercise training often ingest large quantities of protein and carbohydrate after cessation of exercise (i.e. traditional 'weight gainers') to augment net muscle protein accretion. Coingestion of carbohydrate during post-exercise recovery has been shown to improve net leg amino acid balance [3], which has been attributed to the concomitant increase in circulating plasma insulin concentrations [4]. In accordance, elevated plasma insulin levels can increase net muscle protein anabolism in vivo in humans [32, 33]. However, insulin should not be regarded as a primary regulator of muscle protein synthesis as insulin exerts only a modest effect on muscle protein synthesis in the absence of elevated amino acid concentrations. In a recent attempt to assess whether carbohydrate coingestion is required to maximize post-exercise muscle protein synthesis, we observed no additional benefit of the coingestion of either a small or large amount of carbohydrate on post-exercise muscle protein synthesis rates under conditions where ample protein is ingested [11]. Though carbohydrate coingestion does not seem to be required to maximize post-exercise muscle protein synthesis rates, it is likely that some carbohydrate can attenuate the post-exercise rise in muscle protein breakdown rate, thereby improving net protein balance [3, 4]. Furthermore, as muscle glycogen content can be reduced by 30–40% following a single session of resistance type exercise [34], some carbohydrate coingestion may be preferred when these athletes wish to allow full muscle glycogen repletion to maintain optimum exercise capacity.

Timing of Dietary Protein Ingestion

Besides the amount and type of protein ingested, the timing of protein ingestion seems to represent an important factor in stimulating post-exercise muscle anabolism. Levenhagen et al. [35] reported an improved post-exercise net protein balance after consuming a supplement that contained protein, carbohydrate and fat immediately after cessation of exercise as opposed to 3 h later. Furthermore, recent studies suggest that carbohydrate and protein coingestion prior to and/or during exercise may further augment post-exercise muscle protein accretion [16, 36]. Tipton et al. [16] showed that amino acid ingestion prior to, as opposed to after, exercise further augments net muscle protein accretion during subsequent recovery. The stimulating effect of protein or amino acid supplementation prior to exercise on muscle protein synthesis after exercise has been attributed to a more rapid supply of amino acids to the muscle during the acute stages of post-exercise recovery. However, it could also be speculated that protein ingestion prior to and/or during resistance type exercise already stimulates muscle protein synthesis during exercise, thereby creating a larger time frame for muscle protein synthesis to be elevated. In a recent study, we confirmed that coingestion of protein with carbohydrate before and during 2 h of intermittent resistance type exercise stimulates muscle protein synthesis during

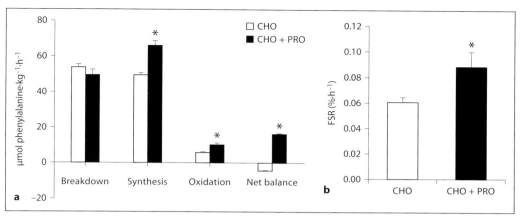

Fig. 2. Protein ingestion prior to and during resistance type exercise stimulates muscle protein synthesis during exercise. **a** Whole-body protein breakdown, synthesis, and oxidation rate as well as net protein balance. **b** FSR of mixed muscle protein during exercise conditions following carbohydrate (CHO) or CHO plus protein (CHO + PRO) ingestion. Values represent means ± SEM. Asterisk denotes significant difference vs. CHO. Figure reproduced from Beelen et al. [36].

exercise [36]. It was speculated that the observed impact of protein coingestion on mixed muscle protein synthesis during exercise is restricted to intermittent, resistance type exercise activities [36]. It remains to be determined if protein ingestion before and/or during exercise also increases muscle protein synthesis during more continuous, endurance type, exercise. Preliminary findings in our lab seem to indicate that even during moderate intensity endurance type exercise muscle protein synthesis rates are stimulated in the working muscle by protein coingestion prior to and during exercise [unpubl. obs.]. More work is needed to address the relevance of the potential to stimulate muscle protein synthesis during as opposed to only after exercise.

Acute versus Long-Term Anabolic Response

Sports nutrition research has traditionally focused on the acute ergogenic properties of various nutritional compounds and/or products. However, the importance of chronic nutritional manipulation to augment the adaptive response to exercise training is receiving increasing attention. The applicability of specific nutritional interventions to improve post-exercise recovery represents a major factor allowing the athlete to maintain performance capacity as well as to improve the adaptive response to more prolonged exercise training. In this regard, more studies are warranted to assess the adaptive response to an acute bout and/or successive bouts of exercise in a setting representative of real-life conditions. Most recovery studies have assessed the impact of nutritional intervention on muscle protein synthesis following a single bout of exercise performed in an overnight fasted state. The latter is not representative of exercise training or competition in which athletes generally practice standard pre-competition dietary guidelines. In addition, most recreational athletes exercise in the evening and have dinner before or after exercise training. In this respect, the benefits of post-exercise nutrition remain largely uninvestigated.

What is the impact of protein and/or amino acid ingestion following exercise on subsequent overnight recovery? For obvious methodological considerations post-exercise muscle reconditioning has hardly been studied during overnight sleep. Recently, we evaluated the impact of exercise performed in the evening on muscle protein synthesis during subsequent overnight recovery [37]. We observed an increase in muscle protein synthesis during the first few hours of post-exercise recovery when protein was being ingested. However, muscle protein synthesis rates during subsequent overnight sleep were unexpectedly low, with values being even lower than most basal, postabsorptive values. Clearly, many people misinterpret the outcome of classic studies like Phillips et al. [2] by suggesting that the post-exercise increase in muscle protein synthesis rate persists for up to 48 h. In accordance, Moore et al. [38] recently reported much greater post-exercise muscle protein synthesis rates after 3 compared with 5 h of post-exercise recovery in the fed state. Clearly, though post-exercise protein ingestion stimulates muscle protein synthesis during the acute stages of post-exercise recovery, these muscle protein synthesis rates are not maintained during subsequent overnight recovery and/or other conditions where amino acid availability is particularly low. Clearly, more research is required to determine the impact of nutrition on post-exercise overnight recovery.

So far, most work in the field aims to establish the impact of nutritional intervention on muscle protein accretion during the acute stages of post-exercise recovery. However, it should be noted that dietary interventions that optimize post-exercise muscle protein accretion do not necessarily translate into a more successful skeletal muscle adaptive response following more prolonged exercise training. Though a discussion on this topic would be beyond the scope of this review, it is evident that numerous intrinsic and extrinsic factors are responsible for orchestrating the long-term skeletal muscle adaptive response to exercise training, and we need to establish the impact of nutrition on these various processes. Specifically designed sports nutrition will have a major impact on optimizing the more prolonged adaptive response to one or several successive bouts of exercise. With regard to the application of protein and/or amino acids, it seems evident that differences in amino acid composition and specific differences in digestion and absorption kinetics would be of great relevance here. As a consequence, more specific designer proteins or protein mixtures will be defined and applied in more individualized sports recovery nutrition, with specificity regarding the type, intensity, duration, and frequency of exercise and optimized for the concomitant priorities set for post-exercise recovery and subsequent muscle tissue reconditioning.

Conclusion

Protein ingestion following either resistance and/or endurance type exercise activities can be used as an effective nutritional strategy to inhibit protein breakdown, stimulate muscle protein synthesis and, as such, augment net muscle protein accretion. The latter has been suggested to lead to a more efficient adaptive response to each successive exercise bout, resulting in improved muscle tissue reconditioning. Whey protein seems most effective in stimulating muscle protein synthesis during acute post-exercise recovery: this is attributed to its rapid digestion and absorption kinetics and specific amino acid composition. About 20 g protein should be provided during and/or immediately after each exercise bout to allow maximum post-exercise muscle protein synthesis rates. Coingestion of large amounts of carbohydrate or free leucine do not further augment post-exercise muscle protein synthesis rates when ample protein is already ingested. Most research has assessed the impact of nutrition on acute post-exercise recovery, with exercise being performed in the morning following an overnight fast. The latter is hardly in line with normal everyday practice, where exercise is generally performed in the evening merely a few hours after the last meal. Future research should focus on the relevance of the acute anabolic response following exercise to optimize the skeletal muscle adaptive response to more prolonged exercise training.

References

1 Chesley A, MacDougall JD, Tarnopolsky MA, et al: Changes in human muscle protein synthesis after resistance exercise. J Appl Physiol 1992;73:1383–1388.
2 Phillips SM, Tipton KD, Aarsland A, et al: Mixed muscle protein synthesis and breakdown after resistance exercise in humans. Am J Physiol 1997;273:E99–E107.
3 Borsheim E, Cree MG, Tipton KD, et al: Effect of carbohydrate intake on net muscle protein synthesis during recovery from resistance exercise. J Appl Physiol 2004;96:674–678.
4 Roy BD, Tarnopolsky MA, MacDougall JD, et al: Effect of glucose supplement timing on protein metabolism after resistance training. J Appl Physiol 1997;82:1882–1888.

5 Biolo G, Maggi SP, Williams BD, et al: Increased rates of muscle protein turnover and amino acid transport after resistance exercise in humans. Am J Physiol 1995;268: E514–E520.
6 Fujita S, Rasmussen BB, Cadenas JG, et al: Effect of insulin on human skeletal muscle protein synthesis is modulated by insulin-induced changes in muscle blood flow and amino acid availability. Am J Physiol Endocrinol Metab 2006;291:E745–E754.
7 Biolo G, Tipton KD, Klein S, Wolfe RR: An abundant supply of amino acids enhances the metabolic effect of exercise on muscle protein. Am J Physiol 1997;273:E122–E129.

8 Tipton KD, Gurkin BE, Matin S, Wolfe RR: Nonessential amino acids are not necessary to stimulate net muscle protein synthesis in healthy volunteers. J Nutr Biochem 1999;10: 89–95.

9 Borsheim E, Tipton KD, Wolf SE, Wolfe RR: Essential amino acids and muscle protein recovery from resistance exercise. Am J Physiol Endocrinol Metab 2002;283: E648–E657.

10 Rasmussen BB, Tipton KD, Miller SL, et al: An oral essential amino acid-carbohydrate supplement enhances muscle protein anabolism after resistance exercise. J Appl Physiol 2000;88:386–392.

11 Koopman R, Beelen M, Stellingwerff T, et al: Co-ingestion of carbohydrate with protein does not further augment post-exercise muscle protein synthesis. Am J Physiol Endocrinol Metab 2007;293:E833–E842.

12 Koopman R, Wagenmakers AJ, Manders RJ, et al: Combined ingestion of protein and free leucine with carbohydrate increases postexercise muscle protein synthesis in vivo in male subjects. Am J Physiol Endocrinol Metab 2005;288:E645–E653.

13 Miller SL, Tipton KD, Chinkes DL, et al: Independent and combined effects of amino acids and glucose after resistance exercise. Med Sci Sports Exerc 2003;35: 449–455.

14 Tipton KD, Elliott TA, Cree MG, et al: Stimulation of net muscle protein synthesis by whey protein ingestion before and after exercise. Am J Physiol Endocrinol Metab 2007;292:E71–E76.

15 Tipton KD, Ferrando AA, Phillips SM, et al: Postexercise net protein synthesis in human muscle from orally administered amino acids. Am J Physiol 1999;276: E628–E634.

16 Tipton KD, Rasmussen BB, Miller SL, et al: Timing of amino acid-carbohydrate ingestion alters anabolic response of muscle to resistance exercise. Am J Physiol Endocrinol Metab 2001;281:E197–E206.

17 Howarth KR, Moreau NA, Phillips SM, Gibala MJ: Coingestion of protein with carbohydrate during recovery from endurance exercise stimulates skeletal muscle protein synthesis in humans. J Appl Physiol 2009; 106:1394–1402.

18 Levenhagen DK, Carr C, Carlson MG, et al: Postexercise protein intake enhances whole-body and leg protein accretion in humans. Med Sci Sports Exerc 2002;34:828–837.

19 Gibala MJ: Protein metabolism and endurance exercise. Sports Med 2007;37:337–340.

20 Moore DR, Robinson MJ, Fry JL, et al: Ingested protein dose response of muscle and albumin protein synthesis after resistance exercise in young men. Am J Clin Nutr 2009; 89:161–168.

21 Tipton KD, Elliott TA, Cree MG, et al: Ingestion of casein and whey proteins result in muscle anabolism after resistance exercise. Med Sci Sports Exerc 2004;36:2073–2081.

22 Wilkinson SB, Tarnopolsky MA, Macdonald MJ, et al: Consumption of fluid skim milk promotes greater muscle protein accretion after resistance exercise than does consumption of an isonitrogenous and isoenergetic soy-protein beverage. Am J Clin Nutr 2007;85:1031–1040.

23 Koopman R, Verdijk L, Manders RJ, et al: Co-ingestion of protein and leucine stimulates muscle protein synthesis rates to the same extent in young and elderly lean men. Am J Clin Nutr 2006;84:623–632.

24 Elliot TA, Cree MG, Sanford AP, et al: Milk ingestion stimulates net muscle protein synthesis following resistance exercise. Med Sci Sports Exerc 2006;38:667–674.

25 Tang JE, Moore DR, Kujbida GW, et al: Ingestion of whey hydrolysate, casein, or soy protein isolate: effects on mixed muscle protein synthesis at rest and following resistance exercise in young men. J Appl Physiol 2009; 107:987–992.

26 Fouillet H, Mariotti F, Gaudichon C, et al: Peripheral and splanchnic metabolism of dietary nitrogen are differently affected by the protein source in humans as assessed by compartmental modeling. J Nutr 2002; 132:125–133.

27 Boirie Y, Dangin M, Gachon P, et al: Slow and fast dietary proteins differently modulate postprandial protein accretion. Proc Natl Acad Sci U S A 1997;94:14930–14935.

28 Dangin M, Boirie Y, Garcia-Rodenas C, et al: The digestion rate of protein is an independent regulating factor of postprandial protein retention. Am J Physiol Endocrinol Metab 2001;280:E340–E348.

29 Dangin M, Guillet C, Garcia-Rodenas C, et al: The rate of protein digestion affects protein gain differently during aging in humans. J Physiol 2003;549:635–644.

30 Koopman R, Crombach N, Gijsen AP, et al: Ingestion of a protein hydrolysate is accompanied by an accelerated in vivo digestion and absorption rate when compared with its intact protein. Am J Clin Nutr 2009;90: 106–115.

31 Koopman R, Verdijk LB, Beelen M, et al: Co-ingestion of leucine with protein does not further augment post-exercise muscle protein synthesis rates in elderly men. Br J Nutr 2008;99:571–580.

32 Gelfand RA, Barrett EJ: Effect of physiologic hyperinsulinemia on skeletal muscle protein synthesis and breakdown in man. J Clin Invest 1987;80:1–6.

33 Hillier TA, Fryburg DA, Jahn LA, Barrett EJ: Extreme hyperinsulinemia unmasks insulin's effect to stimulate protein synthesis in the human forearm. Am J Physiol 1998; 274:E1067–E1074.

34 Koopman R, Manders RJ, Jonkers RA, et al: Intramyocellular lipid and glycogen content are reduced following resistance exercise in untrained healthy males. Eur J Appl Physiol 2006;96:525–534.

35 Levenhagen DK, Gresham JD, Carlson MG, et al: Postexercise nutrient intake timing in humans is critical to recovery of leg glucose and protein homeostasis. Am J Physiol Endocrinol Metab 2001;280:E982–E993.

36 Beelen M, Koopman R, Gijsen AP, et al: Protein coingestion stimulates muscle protein synthesis during resistance-type exercise. Am J Physiol Endocrinol Metab 2008; 295:E70–E77.

37 Beelen M, Tieland M, Gijsen AP, et al: Coingestion of carbohydrate and protein hydrolysate stimulates muscle protein synthesis during exercise in young men, with no further increase during subsequent overnight recovery. J Nutr 2008;138:2198–2204.

38 Moore DR, Tang JE, Burd NA, et al: Differential stimulation of myofibrillar and sarcoplasmic protein synthesis with protein ingestion at rest and after resistance exercise. J Physiol 2009;587:897–904.

Discussion

Dr. Gibala: Relatively few studies have measured muscle protein breakdown (MPB) as it is technically difficult, but in the big picture how much are we missing by not measuring FBR simultaneously with muscle protein synthesis (MPS)? The consensus view is that MPS is the main regulated variable but the different proteins and amino acids can differentially effect the insulin response. What is your view on that?

Dr. van Loon: I think we are missing a significant piece of the puzzle, but as you note there are methodological difficulties, and we cannot accurately measure MPB. A second consideration is that the acute muscle protein anabolic response to exercise and/or food intake may not necessarily reflect what happens over the long term, and chronic transient changes in MPB may contribute considerably to the more prolonged adaptive response to exercise. I feel that protein breakdown is of even greater relevance over the first few days following exercise to allow the reconditioning process to occur. If we look at satellite cell activation and differentiation we see a large number of satellite cells appearing in skeletal muscle tissue 1–2 days after exercise. A few days later they have disappeared again, which implies that massive muscle reconditioning has occurred over these days. So, what is happening in that phase? That skeletal muscle adaptive response that occurs between 4 h and 5 days following exercise has not yet received much attention.

Dr. Gibala: Another methodological issue relates to the determination of muscle blood flow. This is also technically difficult to measure, but relatively small differences in flow can have considerable impact on determinations of muscle protein turnover. An example is the paper by Kevin Tipton that received a lot of attention and suggested that protein feeding prior to exercise stimulated a greater rise in MPS, but this was largely attributable to the blood flow measures, if I recall.

Dr. van Loon: The delivery of the amino acids to the muscle is a key factor driving the muscle protein synthetic response to exercise and nutrition. The postprandial rise in circulating insulin stimulates muscle perfusion and, therefore drives the postprandial muscle protein synthetic response. Tipton has reported that protein ingestion prior to exercise may further augment muscle protein synthesis rates during post-exercise recovery. The latter was explained by the fact that protein ingestion prior to exercise allows the ingested amino acids to be available immediately following cessation of exercise. In contrast, when protein is ingested after exercise, it takes about 30 min for the ingested amino acids to become available. More recently, we showed that muscle protein synthesis rates can already be increased during exercise when protein is provided prior to exercise. The latter further increases the window of opportunity during which protein synthesis is increased following exercise. In short, there are various reasons why it might be advantageous to provide protein prior to and/or during exercise. However, the latter should be investigated in a condition where exercise is performed in a postprandial, as opposed to a postabsorptive, state. This would also be of more practical relevance, as no athlete will compete without having breakfast in the morning.

Dr. Gibala: Many different proteins are synthesized inside skeletal muscle. In the interest of time you were not able to get into the issue of protein subfraction responses, but there is some evidence that different fractions (e.g. mitochondrial, myofibrillar) do not respond in the same manner to a given exercise stimuli. Could you comment on this?

Dr. van Loon: It is obvious that different types of exercise affect the synthesis rates of different sets of proteins. Endurance type exercise will have a greater impact on the synthesis rate of mitochondrial proteins, whereas resistance type exercise activity will strongly stimulate the synthesis of myofibrillar protein. Of course, this is mainly driven by the type of exercise that is performed (i.e. endurance versus more resistance type exercise) and not by the timing, type or dosing regimen of protein intake.

Dr. Maughan: You said no athlete starts their training day without breakfast, but many ultra-distance runners won't eat breakfast before they race because they figure that 100 or 200 g of carbohydrate won't make much difference over 10–12 h of exercise. I suspect there will be a few triathletes on race day who take no food before the race. Certainly, some runners and also many swimmers will do at least some early morning training sessions in the fasted state.

Dr. van Loon: Some athletes train and/or compete in a fasted state. However, to optimize the acute muscle protein synthetic response during and/or after exercise, dietary protein is required. How this translates in a more prolonged adaptation to exercise training remains to be assessed.

Dr. Hawley: The protein literature suggests that an absolute amount of protein (20–25 g) is sufficient to maximally stimulate protein synthesis for individuals with a wide range of body masses. But will the needs of a 100-kg person be the same as someone with a 50-kg body mass and less muscle mass? Please explain how that can be.

Dr. van Loon: The amount of muscle tissue that was actually recruited during the exercise session will likely be the most important factor determining the optimum amount of dietary protein that is needed following exercise. However, at this point we can only say that 20 g of protein appears sufficient to maximize MPS during acute post-exercise recovery in young, lean recreational athletes.

Dr. Hawley: Is that because the studies that have been conducted so far have not systematically compared the response of individuals who range in body size, e.g. a 120-kg man versus a 50-kg woman?

Dr. van Loon: Much of the work is based on men with a body mass of around 85 kg, although the range varies. As far as I know, there is presently only one study that has assessed a dose-response relationship between dietary protein ingestion during acute post-exercise recovery. More work is needed to assess the exact dose of protein that would be needed to optimize the (acute) muscle protein synthetic response to exercise in different populations.

Dr. Phillips: I want to ask about the pre-exercise provision of protein in the Tipton study. Can you explain to me why the authors were unable to reproduce these data in a subsequent study?

Dr. van Loon: I do not know. I can only state that we have recently shown that at least part of the effect that was reported by Tipton's first study is attributed to higher muscle protein synthesis rates during exercise following protein ingestion prior to, as opposed to after, exercise.

Dr. Phillips: Are there differences in the post-exercise muscle protein turnover response to different dietary proteins, i.e. whey versus casein versus soy? There is evidence that whey proteins seem most effective in stimulating muscle protein synthesis during acute post-exercise recovery, and this is attributed to its rapid digestion and absorption kinetics and specific amino acid composition.

Dr. van Loon: I think it depends on when you ingest the different proteins. Digestion and absorption kinetics are important, but if you ingest it prior to exercise then digestion and absorption are of less relevance. If you ingest casein only following exercise it will take at least 30–45 min before there is ample amino acid available in the blood. If you ingest it after exercise, it is probably best to take a protein hydrolysate or whey. If you ingest casein hydrolysate following exercise, it will likely be just as good as whey, so the digestion and absorption kinetics are important when you want the amino acids at a certain point of time, and that's preferably even before exercise.

Dr. Phillips: With regard to the effectiveness of leucine, in the manuscript you use the terminology when ample protein is consumed or adequate protein is consumed. What if a suboptimal protein dose is ingested, e.g. 10 g, and I were to add leucine together to the 20 g level that we think is important to saturate the MPS response. Could it then become ergogenic or give you back the same response?

Dr. van Loon: I deliberately used the word ample because I would like some room for the possibility of leucine to attenuate post-exercise muscle protein breakdown. However, when you provide such large amounts of dietary protein, it's more than sufficient to inhibit protein breakdown, at least on a whole body level. Coming back to the leucine, following exercise I don't see any value for additional leucine ingestion. Many authors have suggested that it has an advantage in the elderly in the postabsorptive phase. But during post-exercise recovery, we have found no evidence that additional leucine ingestion is of any benefit to the muscle protein synthetic response to exercise. Moreover, we have not been able to detect any clinical benefits of leucine supplementation in healthy elderly and elderly diabetics following 3 and 6 months of intervention, respectively. So, we can't reproduce the acute effects of leucine in elderly people in long-term interventions. That is also one of the reasons why I question the validity of extrapolating findings from acute studies to predict the long-term effect of that regimen.

Dr. Zemel: I would like to explore the issues that Dr. Phillips raised regarding dose and type. Just to make sure I understand, if you do a dose-response curve, you get a plateau around 20 g of dietary protein after exercise, with 10 g being suboptimal. Also, if you look at different sources of protein, you see that soy tends not to be as effective as milk despite having an identical amount of protein, so the differences must be attributable to something, whether it is digestion, absorption or amino acid composition. However, the rest of the experiments that you showed were performed at this optimum level of protein and then superimposed with or without carbohydrate, with or without leucine, etc. So, I am still having trouble reconciling the difference between milk and soy if it's not leucine or perhaps an insulin response or a combination of factors. Can you comment on that?

Dr. van Loon: We have very limited data regarding the effect of different proteins ingested after exercise, so I have to rely on data from the postabsorptive phase where there is more evidence regarding the response to the ingestion of different doses and types of protein. We have compared casein with casein hydrolysate having exactly the same amino acid composition and with whey which has a higher leucine content but the same digestion and absorption kinetics as the casein hydrolysate. Whey is most effective for stimulating postprandial muscle protein synthesis, but following exercise I don't believe that small differences in the anabolic response to food intake are of much importance. The latter is explained by the fact that the stimulating effect of exercise is much stronger than the impact of small differences on insulin responses or the small amino acid responses that you see in the postprandial phase. And that's also evident from our recent work that shows that 30% more of the ingested protein is used for the de novo muscle protein synthesis when exercise is performed prior to protein ingestion. After exercise, we should be concerned about getting ample protein in time; the type of protein is likely to be of less relevance at that stage.

Dr. Zemel: I am puzzled about the acute protein signaling responses and how this correlates with long-term adaptation. You showed the only study where there is any relationship between the acute protein synthesis response and the long-term effect on hypertrophy. How good is protein synthesis after exercise as a marker of hypertrophy?

Dr. van Loon: That's a great question, and I can only say that so far every study shows that if you ingest protein following exercise you have a tremendous increase in net balance and a tremendous increase in protein synthesis. However, I would challenge everybody here to look through the literature and find studies that show that protein supplementation following exercise promotes net muscle protein gain more than not supplementing additional protein. The evidence for the additional benefits of protein supplementation to augment muscle hypertrophy is not very strong.

Dr. Maughan: I would go further and say that we need to be cautious in how we interpret an increase in protein synthesis in response to endurance training: endurance training does not result in increased muscle mass. The net change in muscle total protein content is very small and may even be negative. High loads with few repetitions will give you the biggest increases in muscle mass and best strength adaptation. How can we interpret the changes in protein synthesis and breakdown and how do the acute responses to a single exercise bout translate into a long-term training response?

Dr. van Loon: Differences in the impact of exercise and/or nutrition on the acute muscle protein synthetic response do not necessarily translate into long-term adaptive responses following more prolonged intervention. For example, though leucine coingestion has been reported to augment the postprandial muscle protein synthetic response to food intake, we could not detect any measurable changes in muscle mass following 6 months of leucine supplementation in elderly men. The latter is not surprising as there are numerous factors that modulate the long-term adaptive response to exercise and/or nutritional intervention. I would like to invite Dr. Phillips into this discussion since he has recent data showing differences in the acute muscle protein synthetic response to translate successfully into differences in the long-term adaptive response.

Dr. Phillips: We have data in which we tested two paradigms for contraction, 1 set versus 3 sets. We published the acute protein synthetic response, and it clearly showed that it was superior in 3 sets versus 1 set. We have also data that show when you lift at 30% of your maximum voluntary contraction to fatigue you get an equivalent stimulation of protein synthesis as if you were lifting at 90%. And so we have done a training study comparing those two different contraction paradigms, 1 set versus 3 sets or 3 sets of 30% versus work-matched 90%, and the long-term hypertrophy response is predicted by the acute response in both instances.

Dr. Zemel: Are the long-term muscular responses accompanied by similar performance changes?

Dr. Phillips: That's a rather different thing, performance, and we have known for a long time, for example, that the way you train for muscle mass is not necessarily the way you train to optimize performance, especially power.

Dr. Maughan: We should also remember that training does not only affect the muscles: there's a neural component too, and that may account for some of the differences.

Dr. Haschke: I have another comment on protein quality. Most studies are done using common protein sources such as milk, egg, whey, casein and soy, but we don't know whether these are the best proteins under certain circumstances. Using an example from intensive care medicine, it is possible to spike a basic milk product with certain amino acids and then look which amino acid becomes limiting during synthesis. This has allowed the design of products which will come to the market quite soon. The same is true for example for premature babies. The premature baby doubles its body weight in 3 months from 1 to 2 kg. This is a much faster synthesis of protein than occurs in adult life, and we always thought that breast milk would be best. It's not, it serves as the best basis, but if you spike it with amino acids, the infants grow much faster. So, my question is whether you could further improve the protein quality?

Dr. van Loon: I still believe you can improve protein quality and the anabolic response to protein ingestion when it's not in a post-exercise phase. As I mentioned, the exercise response overwhelms almost everything. However, the postprandial muscle protein synthetic response may be further improved by changing dietary protein source, macronutrient composition of a meal, and/or by ingesting specific amino acids or amino acid combinations. But so far, at least in healthy or diabetic elderly, we don't see this being translated to clinical benefits after long-term intervention. However, with intensive care unit patients we see a lot of things happening with infusions over time to attenuate muscle protein breakdown, but in normal consumer nutrition I don't see much evidence for that. Of course, there are always interesting clues from basic nutrition research, e.g.

somebody finds an anabolic response to leucine and then everybody starts working on leucine but many other amino acids tend to get neglected. So, we started screening for the anabolic properties of different amino acids and amino acid combinations. We observed that the rise in the plasma concentrations of these amino acids and/or amino acid combinations shows strong correlations with the muscle protein synthetic response. So, there might be more.

Dr. Maughan: I used to speak to some body builders who told me they would set the alarm clock for every 2 h during the night and get up and have a dose of protein and go back to sleep. Are they doing the right thing or would they be better just getting some sleep?

Dr. van Loon: I think they are doing the right thing, and we have done some work looking at night-time muscle protein synthesis and whether it is limited by the availability of protein. A first study has shown that protein synthesis rates during the night are very low. It has been suggested that amino acids are released from the gut throughout the night, but we didn't find any evidence for that. So, what happens if you provide protein like the body builders do by simply taking a handful of branched chain amino acids and a large protein shake at 3 o'clock in the morning? There might be some rationale for that practice. However, waking up during the night to ingest protein might cause more problems than its proposed benefits, and there are other options to provide protein in a more sustained manner throughout the night.

Dr. Baar: Can I follow up on that? Some studies have looked at long-term amino acid provision and suggested that there is either an insulin resistance or a negative feedback that could have a negative effect and attenuate the response to amino acids. If you take protein every couple of hours or if you maintain a constant high level of amino acids in another way, might that have a negative effect on muscle protein synthesis?

Dr. van Loon: It depends completely on which study you look at. There are also studies that compared spread feeding versus pulse feeding, showing that pulse feeding has a greater anabolic response than spread feeding because nitrogen retention was shown to be much higher. However, these data are based on whole-body nitrogen retention and, as such, might not be representative of the muscle tissue. However, from the other point of view, in many clinical conditions people are being provided with parenteral nutrition constantly, and I am certain that if you apply pulse feeding you don't see the anabolic resistance or the insulin resistance that occurs with continuous feeding. Overall studies suggest that a temporary increase in amino acid provision is the best strategy to promote the anabolic response. This seems superior to continual provision at a more constant level.

Dr. Hawley: I just want to bring it back to the practical, bring it back to the theme of the conference 'Triggers for Adaptation'. I am intrigued with the endurance training response to protein. Should we recommend that instead of just focusing on increasing carbohydrate availability for glycogen resynthesis, endurance athletes should consume 20 g of protein as well?

Dr. van Loon: There is so much that we don't know about. How much protein should be ingested to optimize the acute muscle protein synthetic response to endurance type exercise, and how relevant is it? What kinds of proteins are being synthesized during endurance type exercise? If you believe it is important to stimulate muscle protein synthesis during or immediately after exercise, you should ingest about 20 g of dietary protein. If you do not provide sufficient dietary protein to allow the protein synthesis to occur, you might impair the subsequent adaptive response. But, whether this would have any consequences for the more long-term adaptative response remains to be established. What's the minimum amount of protein required? It may be less than what we are presently providing.

Dr. Gibala: We need more of these long-term studies. They are difficult to do, but that's really what needs to be done.

Dr. Maughan: Measuring performance outcomes is a lot easier to do, and maybe we should do this first: if there is no performance outcome, you don't need to look for a mechanism.

Protein

Maughan RJ, Burke LM (eds): Sports Nutrition: More Than Just Calories – Triggers for Adaptation.
Nestlé Nutr Inst Workshop Ser, vol 69, pp 97–113,
Nestec Ltd., Vevey/S. Karger AG., Basel, © 2011

Effect of Protein, Dairy Components and Energy Balance in Optimizing Body Composition

Stuart M. Phillips[a] · Michael B. Zemel[b]

[a]Exercise Metabolism Research Group – Department of Kinesiology, McMaster University, Hamilton, ON, Canada; [b]The Nutrition Institute, The University of Tennessee, Knoxville, TN., USA

Abstract

Weight loss is achieved through the consumption of a hypoenergetic diet and/or increased energy expenditure through exercise. While weight loss is associated with numerous benefits, the pattern of weight loss in terms of body composition changes is not always studied. In our view, the optimum pattern of weight loss is one in which fat mass is lost and lean mass is preserved. The preservation of lean mass has important consequences due to the role of this tissue in contributing to basal metabolic rate, controlling glycemia, and contributing to lipid oxidation. We also propose that a preservation of lean mass would have important consequences in resisting weight regain after loss. We review dietary practices, including reduced consumption of dietary carbohydrate, consuming higher than recommended dietary protein, with an emphasis on dairy sources, as well as dietary calcium, to accelerate the loss of fat mass during dieting and preserve lean mass. Available evidence suggests that each practice has a highly plausible mechanistic and growing clinical rationale in terms of efficacy in promoting fat mass loss and lean mass retention during a hypoenergetic diet.   Copyright © 2011 Nestec Ltd., Vevey/S. Karger AG, Basel

Introduction

Obesity and leanness are complex genetic traits, with multiple genes interacting to modulate energetic efficiency, including regulation of lipid storage in adipose tissue and lipid oxidation in support of new protein synthesis in skeletal muscle. However, the metabolic pathways operated by these genetic factors may also be modulated by specific nutrients, foods or dietary patterns, providing opportunities for functional foods and ingredients to alter body composition independently of their energy content. Weight loss, however, must depend on either reducing habitual energy intake or/and increasing habitual energy expenditure, or some combination of these two options. Many studies have shown the benefits of both approaches alone and in combination to promote weight loss, favorable blood lipid changes, better glycemic regulation, and a host of other benefits. Nonetheless, the longest-term studies on the efficacy of diet-only weight loss programs have reported that most participants regain their lost weight and continue on an upward trajectory in terms of weight gain [1]. A registry of what have been termed 'successful long-term weight losers' is now maintained and characteristics of those people are being examined [2, 3]. This review will assess the efficacy of certain dietary practices, alone or in combination with programs of exercise, on people's capacity to lose weight and more importantly to affect the pattern of weight loss in terms of body composition. The focus on body composition is important because loss of lean as well as fat mass will have both short- and long-term consequences that may affect a person's capacity to regain weight and affect their metabolic health. The focus of this review is on patterns of dietary macronutrients that appear, at least in short-term studies, to be more effective in promoting loss of fat mass and promoting lean mass retention. We also review the components enriched in dairy, such as calcium, vitamin D (when present as a supplement) and leucine, as important factors in promoting fat mass loss and lean mass retention or accretion.

The relative energy deficit created by dietary energy restriction and/or increased energy expenditure is clearly the primary driver of weight loss, but certain patterns of macronutrients and ingredients might create a generically applicable efficacious approach to weight loss. Dietary patterns may affect the rate and composition of weight loss; however, our recommendations extend beyond the energy deficit. In this review, we focus on weight loss strategies that affect not only the quantity of weight loss but the 'quality' of weight loss. An improved quality of weight loss is defined as being the loss of weight with the highest possible ratio of fat to lean mass loss with the further aim to promote loss of as much visceral body fat as possible. We propose that this weight loss pattern is important for short and long-term metabolic health and possibly aids in resistance to weight regain after loss [4–6]. The measurement of weight loss without focusing on the loss of skeletal muscle as a highly metabolically active tissue is flawed. Skeletal muscle is the largest single contributor to basal metabolic rate (BMR) [7] and its loss during a hypoenergetic period is therefore one of the main reasons why BMR declines with weight loss [8]. A decline in BMR will affect the acute reduction in weight loss and the long-term maintenance of a lower body mass. Weight loss resulting from reduced energy intake will lead to loss of skeletal muscle, which is unlikely to be reclaimed in the absence of resistance exercise to stimulate muscle hypertrophy, resulting in a chronic decline of BMR [9]. Moreover, skeletal muscle is the primary site of postprandial blood

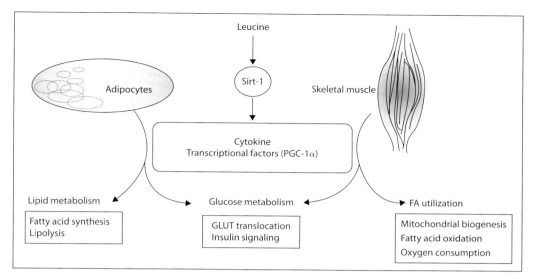

Fig. 1. Effects of leucine on energy partitioning between adipose tissue and skeletal muscle. Leucine stimulates Sirt 1 transcription and activity, resulting in reduced lipid storage and a net increase in lipolysis. Sirt 1 also mediates an increase in muscle mitochondrial biogenesis, fatty acid oxidation and oxygen consumption, and a net increase in insulin sensitivity. Based on data from Sun and Zemel [42].

glucose disposal [10], and thus plays an integral role in regulation of glycemia and risk for type 2 diabetes [10]. Also, due virtually entirely to its mass, skeletal muscle is a significant contributor to lipid oxidation and thus is an important contributor to postprandial lipemia [11] and overall blood lipid regulation [11]. In the light of these roles of skeletal muscle and adipose tissue, it is apparent that weight loss strategies need to protect against loss of skeletal muscle and promote fat, especially visceral fat, loss.

Macronutrient Composition

The macronutrient composition of energy-restricted diets and the influence of these ratios on weight loss remain somewhat controversial. As recently as 2010 in the Dietary Guidelines for Americans the following conclusion was reached: 'There is strong and consistent evidence that when calorie intake is controlled, macronutrient proportion of the diet is not related to losing weight'. (http://www.cnpp.usda.gov/Publications/DietaryGuidelines/2010/DGAC/Report/D-1-EnergyBalance.pdf). An important caveat in this conclusion, however, is in regards to the composition of the weight lost and the failure of the preceding statement to differentiate between the outcomes of subject compliance and diet efficacy [1]. The composition of weight loss with energy-restricted diets is generally 70–80% adipose and 30–20% lean tissue (almost exclusively skeletal muscle) [12]. As stated in the introduction, this pattern of weight loss will influence metabolic function during weight loss. The decline in BMR that accompanies weight loss is a primary reason for the slowed rate of weight loss seen in longer-term programs due to a gradual narrowing of the gap between energy requirement for weight maintenance.

Many weight loss diets set protein at 15% of energy, <30% lipids, and 50–55% carbohydrates, with reductions in dietary fat and increases in dietary fiber being favored. It is reasonable to reduce energy density with this ratio of macronutrients and promote weight loss in the short term, but this diet is associated with low satiety and poor long-term adherence [1, 13, 14]. Emerging evidence suggests that reducing the intake of dietary carbohydrates is critically important for promoting both greater weight loss and greater loss of body fat [13–15]. The mechanisms underpinning this effect are uncertain but may relate to a lower daily blood glucose and insulin levels [16]. Insulin's primary function as a hormone is to promote storage of blood glucose in skeletal muscle and adipose tissue and to inhibit lipolysis and promote triglyceride synthesis and storage [16]. This may explain why a hallmark adaptation to lower carbohydrate diets is a pronounced reduction in circulating triglycerides versus other diets. A proven strategy, and one that is beneficial, is also to reduce not just the total quantity of carbohydrate but also to globally lower the glycemic load of the diet by selecting low glycemic-index (GI) carbohydrate sources [13]. In a weight loss context, such a strategy has been shown to be effective and also results in lowered insulin levels [16] and triglyceridemia [17]. It does need to be highlighted that following lower carbohydrate, lower GI diets may be a problem for endurance athletes seeking to compete since dietary carbohydrate intakes are recommended to be higher to allow full recovery of muscle glycogen stores. While lower total and relative carbohydrate diets appear effective, an important question is what macronutrient should replace the carbohydrate. Diets moderately high (no more than 35% of total energy intake) in protein and modestly restricted in carbohydrate (no less than 35% of total energy intake) and fat may have more beneficial effects on body weight homeostasis and associated metabolic variables [13–17]. Other factors such as dietary omega-3 fatty acids may also be important for weight loss given their impact on satiety and potentially on muscle anabolism. We focus here on moderate-protein diets (30–35% energy at the expense of carbohydrates) and those with low-GI carbohydrates (within the 40% energy).

Increasing protein to higher than the recommended dietary allowance (RDA) levels of 0.8 g protein/kg per day has a beneficial effect on retention of lean mass during hypoenergetic periods of weight loss [13–17]. In fact, in their meta-analysis, Krieger et al. [15] pointed out that in short-term trials (<12 weeks), protein intakes that were 40% higher than the RDA were associated with a 0.60

kg additional fat-free mass retention compared with diets with lower protein intakes. If the trials examined were extended beyond 12 weeks, then this difference grew to a 1.2 kg preservation of lean mass versus lower protein diets. The decrement in lean mass induced by a period of reduced energy intake can also be offset with a resistive exercise component to aid in muscle mass retention [18]. A small handful of studies have also reported that the combination of higher protein consumption and performance of exercise has a synergistic effect in terms of preservation of skeletal muscle mass [18, 19]. An important point is that such a strategy results in less total weight being lost, which may or may not be desirable. A few studies have shown that strength, for example, is preserved during periods of weight loss, and so a consideration for athletes is that if it is weight loss pure and simple that they require then preservation of lean mass may not be concern [20]. However, it is unlikely that such a strategy can continue unabated, and eventually reductions in athletic performance are likely to occur [20]. From the perspective of the metabolic consequences and for the general population, the preservation of lean mass during weight loss would appear of paramount concern.

It is unclear why protein would have a lean mass-sparing effect during weight loss, but it likely relates to the stimulatory effect of protein on muscle protein synthesis (MPS) [21, 22]. The periodic meal-induced stimulation of MPS maintains skeletal muscle mass [21], so it is reasonable to assume that MPS could be stimulated to a greater extent than with a lower protein diet, although there is no direct evidence for this. It is also possible that hypercortisolemia during weight loss would provide a stimulus opposing retention of muscle protein. In men undergoing chronic bed rest with pharmacologically induced elevations in corticoid hormones, a markedly atrophic condition, supplementation with essential amino acids provided some relief against muscle loss [23]. Thus, while it may depend on the extent and duration of the energy deficit and the duration, higher protein diets have been shown to ameliorate loss of lean muscle mass. There may also be a role for higher quality proteins in opposing loss of muscle mass due to the crucial role of leucine in activating the process of MPS and promoting retention of lean mass during hypoenergetic periods [24]. Such a thesis has been proposed and has experimental support in animal models [24], but currently lacks direct experimental evidence in humans. A further extension of this thesis has been provided by Devkota and Layman, who defined the dose of leucine (2.5 g) that is required to stimulate MPS maximally and also provided advice on the meal frequency required to maximally stimulate MPS and thus retain muscle protein [25].

Other mechanisms that have been proposed as to why protein is an effective substitution for dietary carbohydrate relate to protein's satiety-promoting effects, which appear to be greater than those of carbohydrate and fat. In addition, the thermogenic effect of protein consumption has long been known to be the greatest of all macronutrients.

Role of Calcium and Dairy Components

The original concept of calcium and dairy modulation of body composition and weight management emerged as a surprising finding from a clinical trial evaluating the role of dairy in hypertension, with subsequent corroboration via animal studies, cellular studies to provide a mechanistic framework, secondary analysis of clinical studies originally performed to assess skeletal outcomes and finally prospective clinical trials to assess the effects of calcium and dairy foods on adiposity. In the original hypertension study, isoenergetic substitution of yogurt (454 g/day) in the daily diet resulted in a significant 4.9 kg reduction in body fat [26]. This 'anti-obesity' effect of dietary calcium was confirmed in a series of studies conducted in a mouse model of diet-induced obesity (aP-2-agouti transgenic mice [26–28]). These mice responded to low-calcium diets with accelerated weight and fat gain, while high calcium diets markedly inhibited lipogenesis, accelerated lipolysis and fat oxidation, increased thermogenesis and suppressed fat gain with no change in energy intake [26]. Further, when the mice were subjected to modest energy restriction, low-calcium diets inhibited body fat loss, while-high calcium diets markedly accelerated fat loss [26–28]; notably, utilizing dairy as the calcium source without altering macronutrient composition resulted in substantially greater effects compared to calcium carbonate.

Dietary calcium and dairy also alter the partitioning of dietary energy during refeeding following weight loss by obese mice [28]. Although post-obese mice fed low-calcium diets exhibited rapid weight and fat regain, increasing dietary calcium prevented the suppression of lipolysis and fat oxidation that otherwise accompanies energy repletion and instead upregulated skeletal muscle fat oxidation [28], reflecting a repartitioning of energy from storage in adipose tissue to oxidation in skeletal muscle. The result is an increase in metabolic rate that is not compensated for by energy intake. As a result, high calcium diets prevented 50–85% of the weight and fat regain found in the animals fed the low calcium diet, with significantly greater effects found with dairy than with elemental calcium [28].

Mechanisms

The anti-obesity effects of dairy foods include both calcium-dependent and calcium-independent mechanisms. The calcium component appears to be mediated by calcium suppression of calcitrophic hormones and by calcium binding to fatty acids in the gastrointestinal tract, forming soaps and thereby reducing fat absorption [29].

Calcitriol (1,25-dihydroxyvitamin D), released in response to suboptimal calcium intakes, stimulates increases in human adipocyte intracellular Ca^{2+}, while dietary calcium, by virtue of suppressing calcitriol levels, decreases intracellular Ca^{2+} [30]. Increased adipocyte Ca^{2+} signaling stimulates the expression and activity of fatty acid synthase [27, 31, 32], a key regulatory lipogenic gene, resulting in increased lipid synthesis. Elevated intracellular Ca^{2+} also inhibits lipolysis, and the combination of increased lipid synthesis and decreased degradation results in an expansion of adipocyte triglyceride storage [33]. Calcitriol also inhibits the expression of uncoupling protein 2 (UCP2) [34], potentially resulting in increased coupling of mitochondrial energy metabolism to ATP production and increasing the efficiency of adipocyte energy storage, while dietary calcium increases adipose tissue UCP2 expression [34].

Human data support these mechanisms. Suppressing calcitriol with high dairy diets increased lipolysis [35, 36] and caused a 30 g/day (270 kcal/day) increase in fat oxidation in a randomized, controlled crossover study under highly controlled conditions using a whole-room calorimeter [35]. Similarly, long-term (one year) consumption of a dairy-rich high calcium diet resulted in increased fat oxidation responses to meal challenges [37].

Rodent and human studies demonstrate a shift in the distribution of body fat loss on high- versus low-calcium diets during energy restriction, with preferential loss of visceral adipose tissue. Excessive central fat deposition in obesity may result from the greater capacity for local regeneration of active glucocorticoids in the visceral fat depot, which is controlled by the activity of 11β-hydroxysteroid dehydrogenase type 1 (11β-HSD 1) to generate active cortisol. Calcitriol directly upregulates adipocyte 11β-HSD 1 expression and cortisol release and, consequently, correspondingly affects local cortisol levels, indicating a potential role for calcitriol in visceral adiposity [38, 39].

Role of Branched-Chain Amino Acids

Depletion of calcium from milk reduces its anti-obesity efficacy in rodents, but calcium-depleted milk still retains ~50–60% of the anti-obesity bioactivity of intact milk, most of which can be restored by increasing the branched chain amino acid content of a low-calcium/non-dairy diet to the level found in milk or whey [40]. The abundance of leucine in dairy protein is of particular interest, as it plays a pivotal role in translation initiation of protein synthesis and appears to be important for repartitioning of dietary energy from adipose tissue to skeletal muscle [40–42], see fig. 1.

Leucine coordinately regulates lipid metabolism and energy partitioning between adipocytes and skeletal muscle cells [42] by inhibiting energy storage in adipocytes, and stimulating skeletal muscle mitochondrial biogenesis and fatty acid oxidation [42, 43]. These effects may represent a means of supplying the additional metabolic energy necessary to support this additional protein synthesis [42, 43]. These effects resulted in a 33.4 g/day (300 kcal) increase in fat oxidation in sedentary overweight and obese individuals [44].

Clinical Data

Several randomized clinical trials have evaluated the magnitude and significance of this effect in humans. In the initial trial [45], 32 obese adults were maintained on balanced energy deficit diets (500 kcal/day deficit) and randomized to control (0–1 serving/day and 400–500 mg Ca/day supplemented with placebo), high-calcium (control diet supplemented with 800 mg Ca/day), or high-dairy (3–4 servings of dairy foods, primarily milk, total Ca intake of 1,200–1,300 mg/day) diets. The high-calcium diet augmented weight loss by 59%, and the high dairy diet increased it twofold. Fat loss followed a similar trend, with the high-calcium and high-dairy food diets augmenting the fat loss found on the low-calcium diet by 38 and 64%, respectively. This was accompanied by a marked change in the distribution of body fat loss; central (trunk) fat loss represented 19% of the total fat lost on the low-calcium diet, and this was increased to 50 and 66% of the fat lost on the high-calcium and high-dairy diets, respectively [45].

These findings were confirmed in several follow-up randomized clinical trials in Caucasians and African-Americans under conditions of modest energy restriction, and one multi-centre trial with a similar experimental design [46, 47]. In the absence of energy restriction, dairy exerts little effect on body weight but still exerts significant effects on body composition. In the absence of energy restriction, increasing dairy intake resulted in a 5.4% reduction in total body fat and a 4.6% decrease in trunk fat ($p < 0.01$ for both) without any change in body weight while a control group maintained on a low-calcium/low-dairy diet with identical macronutrient composition exhibited no significant changes in total body fat or trunk fat [46]. Data from two long-term large-scale placebo-controlled double-blind intervention trials further support a significant role for calcium in improving adiposity in the absence of energy restriction [48, 49]. This modulation of adiposity by dietary calcium exhibits a threshold effect. Major and colleagues recently demonstrated a highly significant 6 kg weight loss in obese women with low baseline calcium intakes (<600 mg/day), while those consuming higher levels of calcium did not exhibit this effect.

Two studies [50, 51] utilizing a similar design to those noted above [36, 52] found no effect of dairy during energy restriction, but subjects in the higher dairy group in both studies consumed significantly more energy (150–200 kcal/day) than was consumed by subjects in the low-dairy control groups, suggesting that the dairy may have permitted greater energy consumption without adversely affecting body weight. Other clinical trials also support a role for dairy or dairy components in weight management. Whey supplementation resulted in significant augmentation of fat loss accompanied by increases in lean mass in previously sedentary exercising individuals [53] as well as individuals subjected to an energy deficit [54]. Similar effects have been noted in studies of weight regain following energy restriction [55, 56].

Although most clinical trials to date have been conducted in adults, a recent 6-month trial of 120 obese primary school-aged (5.6 + 0.5 years) children with a 3-year follow-up [57] demonstrates that dairy-rich diets contribute significantly to successful weight management, manifested as significant effects on BMI and waist circumference over a 3-year study period.

These effects are also supported by a number of observational studies reporting an inverse relationship between dairy foods and/or dairy components and either body weight or body fat in multiple population groups, including children, young adults and older adults of multiple ethnicities [for a recent review, see 58]. Similar inverse relationships have also been reported in multiple epidemiological studies [58] and secondary analyses of clinical trials originally conducted with other end points [59, 60].

Conclusion

The energy gap between intake and expenditure is the primary determinant of weight loss, but quantitatively minor components may play a major role in weight maintenance in the face of significant daily variation in energy balance. Moreover, focusing only on body weight and not body composition is a flawed approach. Skeletal muscle is the largest tissue contributor to BMR and its preservation is important. Skeletal muscle also plays a large role in postprandial glycemic regulation and lipemia, which highlights the importance of its preservation during weight loss. Thus, hypoenergetic 'strategies' that promote lipolysis and fat mass loss, especially loss of visceral body fat, and incorporate approaches to preserve muscle mass would be desirable over those that blithely address weight loss without regard for composition of that loss. Evidence strongly suggests that certain approaches to weight loss can achieve this pattern. First, fat mass loss is accelerated with a reduction in carbohydrate intake from the population average intake of 55–60% of total energy intake to 40% or less, with particular emphasis on low GI carbohydrates. The main reason for this recommendation has to with maintaining a low systemic insulin concentration, which is a markedly anti-lipolytic hormone. Second, dietary protein would need to be consumed in quantities far higher than the RDA level, making up at least 25–35% of the total hypoenergetic intake. In addition, high-quality proteins rich in branched-chain amino acids, especially leucine, stimulate lean mass retention and fat mass loss. The potential satiety value of protein and the thermogenic response associated with its consumption are further reasons to emphasize the substitution of protein for carbohydrates. Third, calcium intake should be at or above the current adequate intake level of 1,000–1,200 mg daily. Calcium consumption has well-established effects on lipid accretion, lipolysis and oxidation as outlined above, and may have as yet unappreciated effects on appetite and on increasing fecal fat excretion, both of which would enhance the impact of a hypoenergetic diet. Finally, dairy is a good source of two of the highest quality proteins, casein and whey, which are both rich sources of leucine. Dairy is also rich in calcium and other nutrients, which make it an excellent functional food to consume in line with the recommendations above.

References

1 Sacks FM, Bray GA, Carey VJ, et al: Comparison of weight-loss diets with different compositions of fat, protein, and carbohydrates. N Engl J Med 2009;360:859–873.

2 Catenacci VA, Ogden LG, Stuht J, et al: Physical activity patterns in the National Weight Control Registry. Obesity (Silver Spring) 2008;16:153–161.

3 Phelan S, Wyatt H, Nassery S, et al: Three-year weight change in successful weight losers who lost weight on a low-carbohydrate diet. Obesity (Silver Spring) 2007;15: 2470–2477.

4 Avila JJ, Gutierres JA, Sheehy ME, et al: Effect of moderate intensity resistance training during weight loss on body composition and physical performance in overweight older adults. Eur J Appl Physiol 2010; 109:517–525.

5 Warner SO, Linden MA, Liu Y, et al: The effects of resistance training on metabolic health with weight regain. J Clin Hypertens (Greenwich) 2010;12:64–72.

6 Hunter GR, Brock DW, Byrne NM, et al: Exercise training prevents regain of visceral fat for 1 year following weight loss. Obesity (Silver Spring) 2010;18:690–695.

7 Johnstone AM, Murison SD, Duncan JS, et al: Factors influencing variation in basal metabolic rate include fat-free mass, fat mass, age, and circulating thyroxine but not sex, circulating leptin, or triiodothyronine. Am J Clin Nutr 2005;82:941–948.

8 Schoeller DA: The energy balance equation: looking back and looking forward are two very different views. Nutr Rev 2009;67:249–254.

9 Strychar I, Lavoie ME, Messier L, et al: Anthropometric, metabolic, psychosocial, and dietary characteristics of overweight/obese postmenopausal women with a history of weight cycling: a MONET (Montreal Ottawa New Emerging Team) study. J Am Diet Assoc 2009;109:718–724.

10 Holloszy JO: Exercise-induced increase in muscle insulin sensitivity. J Appl Physiol 2005;99:338–343.

11 Karpe F, Ehrenborg EE: PPARdelta in humans: genetic and pharmacological evidence for a significant metabolic function. Curr Opin Lipidol 2009;20:333–336.

12 Weinheimer EM, Sands LP, Campbell WW: A systematic review of the separate and combined effects of energy restriction and exercise on fat-free mass in middle-aged and older adults: implications for sarcopenic obesity. Nutr Rev 2010;68:375–388.

13 Abete I, Astrup A, Martinez JA, et al: Obesity and the metabolic syndrome: role of different dietary macronutrient distribution patterns and specific nutritional components on weight loss and maintenance. Nutr Rev 2010; 68:214–231.

14 Foreyt JP, Salas-Salvado J, Caballero B, et al: Weight-reducing diets: are there any differences? Nutr Rev 2009;67(suppl 1):S99–S101.

15 Krieger JW, Sitren HS, Daniels MJ, Langkamp-Henken B: Effects of variation in protein and carbohydrate intake on body mass and composition during energy restriction: a meta-regression. Am J Clin Nutr 2006;83:260–274.

16 Feinman RD, Fine EJ: Nonequilibrium thermodynamics and energy efficiency in weight loss diets. Theor Biol Med Model 2007;4:27.

17 Layman DK: Protein quantity and quality at levels above the RDA improves adult weight loss. J Am Coll Nutr 2004;23:631S–636S.

18 Layman DK, Evans E, Baum JI, et al: Dietary protein and exercise have additive effects on body composition during weight loss in adult women. J Nutr 2005;135:1903–1910.

19 Mettler S, Mitchell N, Tipton KD: Increased protein intake reduces lean body mass loss during weight loss in athletes. Med Sci Sports Exerc 2010;42:326–337.

20 Rodriguez NR, Di Marco NM, Langley S: American College of Sports Medicine position stand. Nutrition and athletic performance. Med Sci Sports Exerc 2009;41: 709–731.

21 Phillips SM: Protein requirements and supplementation in strength sports. Nutrition 2004;20:689–695.

22 Phillips SM: Dietary protein for athletes: from requirements to metabolic advantage. Appl Physiol Nutr Metab 2006;31:647–654.

23 Paddon-Jones D, Sheffield-Moore M, Urban RJ, et al: The catabolic effects of prolonged inactivity and acute hypercortisolemia are offset by dietary supplementation. J Clin Endocrinol Metab 2005;90:1453–1459.

24 Phillips SM, Tang JE, Moore DR: The role of milk- and soy-based protein in support of muscle protein synthesis and muscle protein accretion in young and elderly persons. J Am Coll Nutr 2009;28:343–354.

25 Devkota S, Layman DK: Protein metabolic roles in treatment of obesity. Curr Opin Clin Nutr Metab Care 2010;13:403–407.

26 Zemel MB, Shi H, Greer B, et al: Regulation of adiposity by dietary calcium. FASEB J 2000;14:1132–1138.

27 Shi H, Dirienzo D, Zemel MB: Effects of dietary calcium on adipocyte lipid metabolism and body weight regulation in energy-restricted aP2-agouti transgenic mice. FASEB J 2001;15:291–293.

28 Sun X, Zemel MB: Calcium and dairy products inhibit weight and fat regain during ad libitum consumption following energy restriction in Ap2-agouti transgenic mice. J Nutr 2004;134:3054–3060.

29 Christensen R, Lorenzen JK, Svith CR, et al: Effect of calcium from dairy and dietary supplements on faecal fat excretion: a meta-analysis of randomized controlled trials. Obes Rev 2009;10:475–486.

30 Zemel MB, Shi H, Greer B, et al: Regulation of adiposity by dietary calcium. FASEB J 2000;14:1132–1138.

31 Claycombe KJ, Wang Y, Jones BH, et al: Transcriptional regulation of the adipocyte fatty acid synthase gene by agouti: interaction with insulin. Physiol Genomics 2000;3: 157–162.

32 Shi H, Norman AW, Okamura WH, et al: 1alpha,25-Dihydroxyvitamin D3 modulates human adipocyte metabolism via nongenomic action. FASEB J 2001;15:2751–2753.

33 Jones BH, Maher MA, Banz WJ, et al: Adipose tissue stearoyl-CoA desaturase mRNA is increased by obesity and decreased by polyunsaturated fatty acids. Am J Physiol 1996;271:E44–E49.

34 Xue B, Greenberg AG, Kraemer FB, Zemel MB: Mechanism of intracellular calcium ([Ca^{2+}]i) inhibition of lipolysis in human adipocytes. FASEB J 2001;15:2527–2529.

35 Melanson EL, Donahoo WT, Dong F, et al: Effect of low- and high-calcium dairy-based diets on macronutrient oxidation in humans. Obes Res 2005;13:2102–2112.

36 Zemel MB, Richards J, Milstead A, Campbell P: Effects of calcium and dairy on body composition and weight loss in African-American adults. Obes Res 2005;13: 1218–1225.

37 Gunther CW, Lyle RM, Legowski PA, et al: Fat oxidation and its relation to serum parathyroid hormone in young women enrolled in a 1-y dairy calcium intervention. Am J Clin Nutr 2005;82:1228–1234.

38 Sun X, Morris KL, Zemel MB: Role of calcitriol and cortisol on human adipocyte proliferation and oxidative and inflammatory stress: a microarray study. J Nutrigenet Nutrigenomics 2008;1:30–48.

39 Morris KL, Zemel MB: 1,25-dihydroxyvitamin D3 modulation of adipocyte glucocorticoid function. Obes Res 2005;13:670–677.

40 Bruckbauer A, Gouffon J, Rekapalli B, Zemel MB: The effects of dairy components on energy partitioning and metabolic risk in mice: a microarray study. J Nutrigenet Nutrigenomics 2009;2:64–77.

41 Ha E, Zemel MB: Functional properties of whey, whey components, and essential amino acids: mechanisms underlying health benefits for active people (review). J Nutr Biochem 2003;14:251–258.

42 Sun X, Zemel MB: Leucine and calcium regulate fat metabolism and energy partitioning in murine adipocytes and muscle cells. Lipids 2007;42:297–305.

43 Sun X, Zemel MB: Leucine modulation of mitochondrial mass and oxygen consumption in skeletal muscle cells and adipocytes. Nutr Metab (Lond) 2009;6:26.

44 Zemel MB, Sun X: Effects of a leucine-containing nutraceutical on fat oxidation in overweight and obese adults. FASEB J 2009; 23:563.36.

45 Zemel MB, Thompson W, Milstead A, et al: Calcium and dairy acceleration of weight and fat loss during energy restriction in obese adults. Obes Res 2004;12:582–590.

46 Zemel MB, Richards J, Milstead A, Campbell P: Effects of calcium and dairy on body composition and weight loss in African-American adults. Obes Res 2005;13: 1218–1225.

47 Zemel MB, Richards J, Mathis S, et al: Dairy augmentation of total and central fat loss in obese subjects. Int J Obes (Lond) 2005; 29:391–397.

48 Zhou J, Zhao LJ, Watson P, et al: The effect of calcium and vitamin D supplementation on obesity in postmenopausal women: secondary analysis for a large-scale, placebo controlled, double-blind, 4-year longitudinal clinical trial. Nutr Metab (Lond) 2010;7:62.

49 Caan B, Neuhouser M, Aragaki A, et al: Calcium plus vitamin D supplementation and the risk of postmenopausal weight gain. Arch Intern Med 2007;167:893–902.

50 Thompson WG, Rostad HN, Janzow DJ, et al: Effect of energy-reduced diets high in dairy products and fiber on weight loss in obese adults. Obes Res 2005;13:1344–1353.

51 Harvey-Berino J, Gold BC, Lauber R, Starinski A: The impact of calcium and dairy product consumption on weight loss. Obes Res 2005;13:1720–1726.

52 Zemel MB, Richards J, Mathis S, et al: Dairy augmentation of total and central fat loss in obese subjects. Int J Obes (Lond) 2005;29: 391–397.

53 Lockwood CM, Moon JR, Tobkin SE, et al: Minimal nutrition intervention with high-protein/low-carbohydrate and low-fat, nutrient-dense food supplement improves body composition and exercise benefits in overweight adults: a randomized controlled trial. Nutr Metab (Lond) 2008;5:11.

54 Frestedt JL, Zenk JL, Kuskowski MA, et al: A whey-protein supplement increases fat loss and spares lean muscle in obese subjects: a randomized human clinical study. Nutr Metab (Lond) 2008;5:8.

55 Ochner CN, Lowe MR: Self-reported changes in dietary calcium and energy intake predict weight regain following a weight loss diet in obese women. J Nutr 2007;137:2324–2328.

56 Zemel MB, Donnelly JE, Smith BK, et al: Effects of dairy intake on weight maintenance. Nutr Metab (Lond) 2008;5:28.

57 Kelishadi R, Zemel MB, Hashemipour M, et al: Can a dairy-rich diet be effective in long-term weight control of young children? J Am Coll Nutr 2009;28:601–610.

58 Zemel MB: Proposed role of calcium and dairy food components in weight management and metabolic health. Phys Sportsmed 2009;37:29–39.

59 Davies KM, Heaney RP, Recker RR, et al: Calcium intake and body weight. J Clin Endocrinol Metab 2000;85:4635–4638.

60 Shahar DR, Schwarzfuchs D, Fraser D, et al: Dairy calcium intake, serum vitamin D, and successful weight loss. Am J Clin Nutr 2010;92:1017–1022.

Discussion

Dr. Zemel: I'd like to see us bring back the issues related to performance for just a minute. As you pointed out, when you lose weight, about 30% of what you lose is lean mass. However, overweight people have significantly more lean mass to begin with, as a result of moving their extra weight through their activities of daily living. So, using the strategies that you have described, including higher protein, lower carbohydrate and higher dairy to retain lean mass while losing body fat, would you suggest that post-obese individuals who have successfully gone through a program like this might have improved performance as a result of greater lean mass when compared to individuals who maintained their ideal body weight throughout?

Dr. Phillips: The body weight change in our IDEAL study, was lowest on the high dairy protein group because they gained muscle as they lost fat, so the net weight change is about 100% fat loss, and I agree with your point. Whether performance correlates with that, I can't say. However, many of these very big people cycle through repeated weight loss programs, with loss of skeletal muscle mass each time, and they never fully reclaim it back. As a result, their resting metabolic rate begins to decline and they have an even tougher time losing weight.

Dr. Zemel: When we are talking about macronutrients, as we have up until now, it's very easy to keep in mind that we are talking about nutrition. When we start talking about micronutrients, whether we are talking about leucine or calcium, there is a tendency to forget that we are talking about nutrition and attribute a degree of magical pharmacology to the micronutrient that we are talking about, which brings me back to the nice comments you gave about the work from Angelo Tremblay's lab in which he showed a much greater effect in those with low calcium levels as opposed to those who had fully replete levels of calcium intake. This may not be a calcium-sensing issue but instead simply that you are correcting a suboptimal intake.

Dr. Phillips: Interestingly, he reported a similar phenomenon when women were given a multivitamin during a weight loss program, so maybe it's because they had a poor dietary pattern to start with and that this correction can improve their weight loss pattern. So, I am in full agreement, but I struggle with that from a mechanistic standpoint.

Dr. McLaughlin: We should remember that the gut is a nutrient-sensing organ and the gut endocrine system plays a big role in satiety. There is some recent evidence suggesting that the same calcium receptor that's expressed in the parathyroid may also be expressed in gut endocrine cells, so the gut should be able to sense the luminal calcium content.

Dr. Lang: I am puzzled about vitamin D. We have just learned that $1,25(OH)_2D$ stimulates calcium entry and that this inhibits lipolysis, yet you add vitamin D to milk which would increase $1,25(OH)_2D$.

Dr. Phillips: No, what we add is vitamin D_3 (cholecalciferol), the same fortified form of vitamin D that is in the milk. It doesn't change the active metabolite (1,25-dihydroxy-D) levels.

Dr. Zemel: Remember that most North Americans have either deficient or suboptimal levels of vitamin D as measured by 25-hydroxy vitamin D levels. The other thing is that below 30 ng per ml as you increase dietary vitamin D and increase 25-hydroxy vitamin D you feed back on PTH and lower PTH levels, so those higher levels of 25-hydroxy vitamin D lead to a reduction, not an increase, in 1,25-D, so it's a paradoxical decrease.

Dr. Phillips: I didn't show data here, but we conducted a study over 18 months, and we found that while these women were not deficient, they were definitely not fully sufficient. This is a grey zone, and may be a conundrum for the dairy industry to talk about dairy being a good source of vitamin D because the level of fortification of dairy products in Canada is such that 3 servings gives you 200 IU of vitamin D which is the current recommended intake. However, this may be 5- to 10-fold less than it should be (1,000 or 2,000 IU), and even with 6 servings of dairy those women were getting only about 450 IU of vitamin D. But the parathyroid hormone levels went down in the high dairy group, although we saw no change in 25-hydroxy-D.

Dr. van Loon: Do the glucocorticoids stimulate calcium entry in adipocytes?

Dr. Zemel: I don't know if I can answer the question of whether they stimulate calcium entry, but the adipocyte does have an 11-β-hydroxysteroid dehydrogenase, so it does make its own cortisol. This is an odd relationship between glucocorticoids and $1,25(OH)_2D$, with a feed forward mechanism between the product of 11-β-HSD (cortisol) and the vitamin D receptor in the adipocyte. So 1,25 D stimulates 11-β-HSD to produce cortisol, cortisol then upregulates the vitamin D receptor in the adipocyte with this positive feedback. That's not a direct answer but that's as much as I know.

Dr. Hawley: With those elderly or aging women, you find an alteration of muscle mass loss, so what happens in athletes who want to lose fat mass while retaining a high energy expenditure, with protein intake in excess of 50% of dietary energy? Would you expect supplementation with dairy to have any effect on maintenance of muscle mass during energy restriction in athletes under these conditions?

Dr. Phillips: Correcting low calcium intakes will probably result in a loss of more fat mass in those athletes. The retention of lean mass comes from a combination of two signals: provision of protein at regular levels, and resistive/weight-bearing exercise. While those in the high dairy protein group gained lean mass, we found that the women that gained the most lean mass lost the least amount of fat mass. My interpretation of that is that they were the ones who did not comply with the diet, so the closer you get to energy balance or energy surfeit, the more lean mass you gain, it makes sense. What you can't get are absolutely huge changes; a trainer reported he gained 15 pounds and he lost 15 pounds of fat, but I don't believe it. I think you can shift it a little bit, and so I think you can do it in athletes, but the closest we have is the data from the novice trainers in our milk study in terms of their body composition and then the women in that situation.

Dr. Hawley: The difference is that their total protein intake is still way beyond what is needed. In the endurance-trained athlete with an energy intake of 15 or 17 MJ per day who tries to reduce fat mass, further increasing protein content doesn't seem to be physiologically relevant. So, what would you advise for an athlete? To lose the least amount of muscle mass during periods of energy intake restriction?

Dr. Phillips: Our women in this study ended up with around 1.6 g of protein per kg per day, which is twice the RDA. Most endurance athletes, even at 15% protein, come close to these intakes because of their large energy expenditure, but what becomes more important is then the timing of the protein intake. Small amounts of protein immediately after exercise might prevent that catabolic loss of muscle.

Dr. Gibala: Your data are very important because many people believe that exercise stimulates AMPK, which feeds back to inhibit mTOR; a little bit of protein apparently will overcome that.

Dr. Baar: I don't think that there is any doubt that AMP kinase and mTOR activity can go up at the same time. It only becomes an issue when you get to the elite level, where small changes make the difference: there it becomes an issue, but it is not important for average people. In extreme conditions where you use proper nutrition, the mTOR interaction is minimized.

Dr. Hawley: The IDEAL study data are very compelling and it's interesting to know that the ratio of energy restriction to exercise was heavily biased towards restriction of energy intake.

Dr. Phillips: What I initially wanted to do was to have these women come in 5 days a week and walk around our indoor track at a specified pace. However, my graduate student said we have to give them some flexibility, so we gave them a device called the body media armband that senses skin temperature, heat flux, and has a bi-axial accelerometer and that's programmed to count 250 cal; it counts down and it's a great feedback, but it's independent of exercise. I agree with you and would have liked to have gone a little bit heavier in terms of the exercise, but we were very worried about adherence. In retrospect, adherence to the diet was not good while the adherence to the exercise was exceptional. The women in the high dairy group gained more strength in a few selected exercises; they didn't gain much strength, as they were training only two days a week, but it was greater in that group. In an athletic population you could probably hit the exercise harder, but the dietary restriction tends to contribute to the fat loss. I do think that the reduction in carbohydrate at the right phase of their training cycle is important for mediating fat loss.

Dr. Gibala: Do you think that adherence to the diet will continue? I know some individuals found the high dairy diet to be tough.

Dr. Phillips: With 90 women from diverse ethnic backgrounds, we expected some lactose intolerance, and 46 women came into the study and said they were lactose intolerant. However, only one woman had to drop because of GI symptoms, so lactose intolerance was not a big issue. At the end of the study, we gave them an enormous questionnaire to ask them to rate their perceived adherence to the diet: we knew their exercise adherence because they had to come in to the gym to train. We did look at some body image issues, and the differences between the diets were fairly small, but the exercise efficacy, what they felt they could do, was greatly enhanced. The diet not as much, but they definitely felt they could stick with the exercise after this.

Dr. Haschke: A short comment on milk protein. We had a Nestlé Nutrition Workshop on the value of milk because the company is probably the biggest producer of milk in the world, so we have a high interest in the value of milk. A group from Frankfurt and Offenbach showed that milk protein per se has a very unfavorable insulinogenic index. It stimulates insulin secretion more than all other reference proteins used. They showed in animal experiments that this is a predisposing factor to insulin resistance, and they have good epidemiological data now that this might be associated in risk groups, those who are obese, with the development of type 2 diabetes. There was a response from another group from Puna, India, where 40–50% of people have diabetes type 2 and their protein source is milk because in that area people are 70–80% vegetarians, so their only protein intake from animal sources is milk. If you are proposing very high intake of milk protein for at-risk groups, I think they should be evaluated first.

Dr. Phillips: I completely dispute that data. The most recent meta-analyses have actually shown that it's entirely the opposite, that consumption of milk in dairy products actually reduces the incidence of type 2 diabetes and reduces the incidence particularly of metabolic syndrome, and so I am not sure that I put any stock in those data.

Dr. Haschke: I am neutral because I just report here what was said and has been published. The fact that the milk protein is more insulinogenic than the other ones is clear: this cannot be disputed. The other things, the long-term effects, I agree with you, this has to be shown.

Dr. Phillips: The consensus on this is that the health benefits of milk and dairy consumption are far from negative; so, as an isolated protein I would agree with the insulin response, but in the context of consuming dairy products as a food, there is no difference, and so if I wanted to compare the insulin response of consumption of milk with consumption of a soft drink, for example.

Dr. Haschke: This is a different story, one is protein and the other one is carbohydrate. I am just focusing on the protein quality. Excess of one protein might not be so good, but in balance I think it's adequate and should be consumed. Nobody is against milk for the healthy population, but I just wanted to bring this up as a caveat that we should not go in one direction without being sure.

Dr. van Loon: We should also look at the mechanism. We spent 10 years in looking at how to optimize the insulinotropic response of amino acids and specific proteins. Proteins with a high leucine content which are easily digested and absorbed give a very high insulin response, especially when coingested with carbohydrates. If you add protein or add the right protein to each meal, you actually get a greater glucose disposal capacity and a reduced glycemic response; we have done this and improved glycemic control in diabetics, for example.

Dr. Haschke: Glycemic control is no problem: milk has a very low glycemic index, but it has nothing to do with the insulinogenic index.

Dr. van Loon: But if you take a glass of milk with a high carbohydrate meal your subsequent glycemic response will be improved simply by stimulating the insulinotropic potential of the meal, and that is advantageous.

Dr. Zemel: Milk protein by itself is an insulinotropic agent, without a doubt, but when you substitute milk protein for other proteins in a meal while keeping macronutrients constant, insulin resistance index actually goes down. This was reported in both cohort and randomized clinical trials. For example, 10-year data from the CARDIA study show each of the elements of the insulin resistance syndrome going down, including an improvement in insulin sensitivity.

Dr. Haschke: Are these effects from milk and milk proteins?

Dr. Phillips: It is dairy products. That's the whole point; it's part of an entire diet. In fact, if you want to talk about the glycemic load of the diets, they are about the same, but I can tell you that the insulin sensitivity index in the high dairy protein group improved the most.

Dr. Montain: The military have a different challenge. Soldiers go out on a patrol and are moving about so much that it's hard to get enough food so they tend to lose weight during that period of time; then they come back to the base and have a chance to recover. But often they lose weight and they complain that they have lost strength and ability to work. Evidently, their recovery time is not long enough or they eat poorly during that period of time. What strategy would you recommend?

Dr. Phillips: My understanding is that soldiers practice all kinds of dietary habits, with some eating rushed throughout the day in small amounts, and some sitting down to eat all at once. Obviously, we would advocate for a good percentage of their energy coming from protein and lower glycemic index carbohydrates as opposed to coming from simple sugar. From the standpoint of when they should eat and how often, it comes back to an optimal strategy of consuming a bolus of protein close to 20 g at a time. Outside of that, I am not sure I can do much more. Obviously, they have got a lot of other things going on, and I am not so sure that the loss in strength that they talk about is as much lean mass loss as it is a psychological issue, but maybe that's something from a neurotransmitter standpoint that is mediated by protein as well.

Dr. Montain: What about their recovery then?

Dr. Phillips: There are three masters you have to serve: rehydration, glycogen restoration and repair and adaptation. If you feed a soldier, I don't know whether adaptation is important but definitely repair for a damaged muscle or ligaments requires some substrate. I don't know what the optimal prescription is, but it would certainly be similar to an athlete. If it's practical, they should eat as soon as possible, because recovery starts from there.

Dr. van Loon: If people switch to high protein intake over short periods of time and then switch to very low energy intake, you don't adapt to the situation and that could also cause a massive lean muscle mass loss; nobody has really looked at that, but if you increase protein intake to a very high level for a few weeks and then immediately close it down again you get a different situation.

Dr. Phillips: I think that might be one of our issues.

Dr. Maughan: Elite strength-trained athletes who have qualifying competitions and eat very high amounts of protein up to those qualifying competitions tell us that when they then ease off, they lose enormous amounts of muscle mass in the space of a week or two. This fits with Joe Millward's adaptive metabolic demands model, because they have gone from enormously high protein intake to a relatively normal intake.

Dr. Phillips: If you want to preserve muscle mass, you have got to wean yourself off of a high protein intake, there is no question about that. We are talking about consuming protein here probably over and above what we could be able to put into the muscle, and there is no question but it's acting as a satiety signal in a lot of these situations too.

Dr. Burke: What about populations that are athletic or happy to do more exercise than the 250 cal a day; if they are hypoenergetic and want to have a high protein intake, given the insulinemic protection with dairy protein, would you sacrifice some fat and allow more carbohydrate intake so that you have got more fuel requirements replaced?

Dr. Phillips: If you are going to cut down carbohydrate, it's either protein or fat replacement.

Dr. Burke: But if you preserve the protein, could you sacrifice some fat and keep the carbohydrate high and allow more fuel replacement?

Dr. Phillips: Maintaining protein intakes would aid adherence to the diet, because the protein is an important satiety signal.

Dr. Burke: I am keeping the protein the same. I am wondering if it's just fitting around the carbohydrate and if all dairy is the same, and so if are you thinking about cheese or milk where you have got casein versus the whey components, are we going to see the same effect?

Dr. Phillips: The 6 servings of dairy here were 4 servings as fluid skim milk, two of them chocolate flavor, 3 small yoghurts, each as a half serving and a serving of cheese, so it was just dairy but with no attention paid to one type or the other. I don't know whether you get something different from each different type. However, there is difference in satiety signals that come from fluids as opposed to solids, so we thought that it was better to mix it up.

Dr. Burke: If you talk about dairy, is cheese the same as milk and yoghurt?

Dr. Zemel: In our animal studies, we isolate the non-calcium bioactivity to whey, so I wouldn't expect equal benefit from cheese. We have never done a study with cheese only, but where we have given 3 or 4 servings of dairy per day, we would never allow more than one of those servings to be cheese simply because I was concerned about stripping the whey out of the diet. Obviously, when we use milk and yoghurt, we have both the casein and the whey present. So, while we don't have clinical data to answer your question, our animal data indicate that cheese is not the same.

Dr. Maughan: It is well recognized in the farming business that high protein diets are good for weight loss. Cattle with a bit too much fat have difficulty calving, but putting more protein in the feed for 2 weeks can result in a weight loss of 20–30 kg, almost all of it fat. Maybe we can learn something from the farming world.

Water

Maughan RJ, Burke LM (eds): Sports Nutrition: More Than Just Calories – Triggers for Adaptation.
Nestlé Nutr Inst Workshop Ser, vol 69, pp 115–130,
Nestec Ltd., Vevey/S. Karger AG., Basel, © 2011

Effect of Cell Hydration on Metabolism

Florian Lang

Department of Physiology I, University of Tübingen, Tübingen, Germany

Abstract

Prerequisites for cell survival include avoidance of excessive cell volume alterations. Cell membranes are highly permeable to water, which follows osmotic gradients. Thus, cell volume constancy requires osmotic equilibrium across cell membranes. Cells accumulate osmotically active organic substances and compensate their osmolarity by lowering cytosolic Cl^- concentrations. Following cell shrinkage, regulatory cell volume increase is accomplished by ion uptake (activation of Na^+, K^+, $2Cl^-$ cotransport, Na^+/H^+ exchange in parallel to Cl^-/HCO_3^- exchange and Na^+ channels), by cellular accumulation of organic osmolytes (e.g. myoinositol, betaine, phosphorylcholine, taurine) as well as by proteolysis leading to generation of amino acids and glycogenolysis generating glucose phosphate. Following cell swelling, cell volume is restored by ion exit (activation of K^+ channels and/ or anion channels, KCl cotransport, parallel activation of K^+/H^+ exchange and Cl^-/HCO_3^- exchange), release or degradation of organic osmolytes as well as stimulation of protein synthesis and of glycogen synthesis. The activity of cell volume regulatory mechanisms is modified by hormones, transmitters and drugs, which thus influence protein and glycogen metabolism. Moreover, alterations of cell volume modify generation of oxidants and the sensitivity to oxidative stress. Deranged cell volume regulation significantly contributes to the pathophysiology of several disorders such as liver insufficiency, diabetic ketoacidosis, hypercatabolism, ischemia, and fibrosing disease.

Introduction

Avoidance of excessive alterations of cell volume is an obvious prerequisite for cell survival [1]. Undue cell shrinkage or swelling interferes with the integrity of cell membrane and cytoskeletal architecture. Moreover, cell hydration has a profound influence on cytosolic proteins. Proteins and protein-bound water occupy a large fraction of the intracellular space (macromolecular crowding) leaving only little space for free water [1]. Loss or gain of water approaching only a few percent of cell volume thus exerts a profound effect on protein function and cellular performance.

Water channels allow rapid movement of water across the plasma membrane [2], which is driven by osmotic pressure gradients [1]. Hydrostatic pressure gradients across mammalian cell membranes are negligibly low. To achieve cell volume constancy, cells have to accomplish osmotic equilibrium across the cell membrane. If intracellular osmolarity exceeds extracellular osmolarity, water enters following its osmotic gradient and the cell swells. Conversely, if extracellular osmolarity exceeds intracellular osmolarity water exits leading to cell shrinkage [1, 3–7].

Intra- or extracellular osmolarity and thus osmotic equilibrium across the cell membrane are challenged by alterations of extracellular osmolarity, extracellular ion composition, transport across the cell membrane and cytosolic generation or disposal of osmotically active cytosolic components. Cells employ a variety of mechanisms to maintain cell volume constancy, including altered transport across the cell membrane and metabolism. Hormones and mediators may modify the activity of these cell volume regulatory mechanisms and thus influence cell volume sensitive functions. Accordingly, cell volume regulatory mechanisms are an integral part of the signaling mediating cellular effects of hormones and mediators [1].

Following untoward cell swelling, volume regulatory mechanisms decrease intracellular osmolarity and cell volume, thus accomplishing regulatory cell volume decrease. Following cell shrinkage, cell volume regulatory mechanisms increase intracellular osmolarity and cell volume thus accomplishing regulatory cell volume increase [1, 3–7]. Cell volume regulation is most rapidly accomplished by ion transport across the cell membrane [5]. Following cell swelling, cellular ions are released; upon cell shrinkage, ions are accumulated (fig. 1). However, high cytosolic inorganic ion concentrations interfere with the stability of cytosolic proteins and alterations of ion gradients across the cell membrane may interfere with cell function. To circumvent those problems, cells utilize in addition organic osmolytes for osmoregulation [8]. Organic osmolytes are particularly important in kidney medulla with its excessive hypertonicity [9].

In the following paper, cell volume regulatory mechanisms and several factors challenging cell volume constancy will be described. Moreover, the impact of cell volume on metabolism will be briefly reviewed.

Balance of Cytosolic Osmolarity

The cellular accumulation of organic substances, such as amino acids generates cytosolic osmolarity. Osmotic balance across the cell membrane is accomplished by lowering of the cytosolic inorganic ion concentration below that of

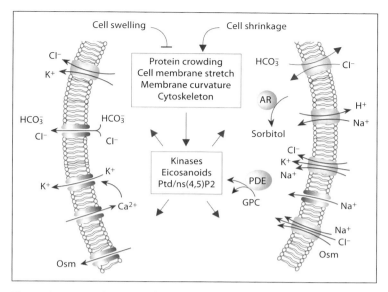

Fig. 1. Major mechanisms of cell volume regulation.

extracellular fluid [1]. To this end, cells extrude Na^+ in exchange for K^+ by the Na^+/K^+-ATPase. The cell membrane is largely impermeable to Na^+ but highly permeable to K^+. The chemical K^+ gradient drives K^+ exit through K^+ channels leading to a cell-negative potential difference across the cell membrane which drives Cl^- exit. The low cytosolic Cl^- concentration outweighs the high concentration of osmotically active organic substances.

The operation of the Na^+/K^+-ATPase and thus the establishment of the ionic gradients require expenditure of energy. Thus, cell volume constancy is challenged by cellular energy depletion, which impairs the function of the Na^+/K^+-ATPase, dissipates the Na^+ and K^+ gradients, depolarizes the cell membrane and leads to cellular accumulation of Cl^- and cell swelling [1]. During ischemia, the cellular K^+ loss leads to increase in extracellular K^+ concentration, which decreases the driving force for K^+ exit and depolarizes the cell further. Moreover, excessive formation and reduced removal of lactate leads to cellular acidification, which in turn stimulates the Na^+/H^+ exchanger and thus augments cellular Na^+ accumulation and cell swelling. The time course of cell swelling during energy depletion depends on the rate of Na^+ entry [1]. In theory, in a completely Na^+ impermeable cell, K^+ and Cl^- approach an equilibrium which does not require any expenditure of energy for the maintenance of cell volume constancy. In some cells, energy depletion leads to transient cell shrinkage, preceding the eventual cell swelling. In those cells, the increase in intracellular Na^+ concentration reverses the driving force for the Na^+/Ca^{2+} exchanger and thus leads to Ca^{2+}

entry, activation of Ca^{2+}-sensitive K^+ channels and/or Cl^- channels, KCl exit and thus cell shrinkage.

Regulatory Cell Volume Increase

Following exposure of cells to hypertonic extracellular medium or cellular loss of osmolytes, the cytosolic osmolarity is lower than the extracellular osmolarity, and water exits leading to cell shrinkage. Regulatory cell volume increase in shrunken cells is mainly accomplished by cellular ion uptake [5]. Cell shrinkage triggers activation of the Na^+, K^+, $2Cl^-$ cotransporter and/or of the Na^+/H^+ exchanger in parallel to the Cl^-/HCO_3^- exchanger [5]. H^+ and HCO_3^- extruded by the Na^+/H^+ exchanger and the Cl^-/HCO_3^- exchanger, respectively, are replenished in the cell from CO_2 via H_2CO_3. The activation of the carriers thus accomplishes NaCl entry. Na^+ accumulated by either Na^+, K^+, $2Cl^-$ cotransport or Na^+/H^+ exchange is pumped out by the Na^+/K^+-ATPase in exchange for K^+. Thus, the transporters eventually accomplish cellular KCl uptake. The two Na^+, K^+, $2Cl^-$ cotransporters NKCC1 and NKCC2 [4] and the Na^+/H^+ exchanger isoforms NHE1, NHE2 and NHE4 are activated, whereas NHE3 is inhibited by cell shrinkage [4].

Regulatory cell volume increase could be further achieved by activation of Na^+ channels and depolarization, which in turn dissipates the electrical gradient for Cl^- and thus leads to Cl^- entry [10]. Some cells inhibit K^+ channels and/or inhibit Cl^- channels upon cell shrinkage to avoid cellular KCl loss [1]. Cell shrinkage is further counteracted by cellular uptake or generation of organic osmolytes, such as sorbitol, myoinositol, betaine, glycerophosphorylcholine (GPC) and taurine [4, 8]. Sorbitol is generated from glucose, a reaction catalyzed by aldose reductase, which is expressed following osmotic cell shrinkage [8]. The expression of the protein is slow and the appropriate sorbitol concentrations are reached only within hours to days. GPC is produced from phosphatidylcholine by a phospholipase A_2 and degraded by a phosphodiesterase. Cell shrinkage interferes with the degradation, thus leading to cellular accumulation of GPC.

Myoinositol (inositol), betaine and taurine are accumulated by the respective Na^+-coupled transporters SMIT, BGT and NCT [4]. The transporters accumulate Na^+ and BGT and NCT Cl^- in parallel to organic osmolytes. Cell shrinkage stimulates and enhances the cellular accumulation of the osmolytes by the expression of the respective transporters. The expression of the transporters is slow and full adaptation requires hours to days. Beyond that, the osmolyte uptake depends on the availability of osmolytes in extracellular fluid.

Cellular concentration of osmotically active amino acids can be accomplished by both, cell volume-sensitive Na^+-coupled transport or degradation of intracellular proteins [1]. Organic osmolytes counteract the destabilizing effects of inorganic ions, organic ions (e.g. spermidine) and urea, as well as the destabilizing effects of heat shock, desiccation and presumably radiation [1].

Regulatory Cell Volume Decrease

Following exposure of cells to hypotonic extracellular fluid or cellular excess of osmolytes, the cytosolic osmolarity is higher than the extracellular osmolarity, and water enters leading to cell swelling. Regulatory cell volume decrease could be accomplished by release of cellular ions by activation of K^+ channels and/or anion channels [10, 11]. Cell volume regulatory K^+ channels include Kv1.3, Kv1.5, Kv4.2,3, KCNE1/KCNQ1,4,5 TWIK1, TASK2/KCNK5, TREK1/KCNK2, TRAAK/KCNK4, intermediate or MaxiK (Kca) [4]. Cell volume regulatory anion channels are ClC-2, ClC-3, phospholemman and bestrophins. The involvement of I_{Cln}, P-glycoprotein (MDR) and CFTR has been a matter of controversy [4, 12]. In any case, several distinct ion channels contribute to cell volume regulation. In some cells, swelling activates unspecific cation channels with subsequent entry of Ca^{2+} and activation of Ca^{2+}-sensitive K^+ channels and/or Cl^- channels [4]. Cell volume regulatory ion exit could be further accomplished by activation of KCl cotransport [4]. In some cells, KCl exits via parallel activation of K^+/H^+ exchange and Cl^-/HCO_3^- exchange. The H^+ and HCO_3^- thus taken up by those transporters react via H_2CO_3 to CO_2 which easily passes the cell membrane and is thus not osmotically relevant.

Cell swelling stimulates the exit of GPC, sorbitol, inositol, betaine and taurine [13]. The mechanisms mediating the release of organic osmolytes are ill defined and may involve several transporters and/or channels in parallel.

Influence of Cell Volume on Metabolism

Cell volume regulates a wide variety of functions including metabolism (fig. 2). For instance, cell shrinkage stimulates proteolysis and inhibits protein synthesis. The amino acids generated by net protein degradation are osmotically more active than the respective proteins. Accordingly, prevailing proteolysis generates cellular osmolarity. Conversely, cell swelling stimulates protein synthesis and inhibits proteolysis and glycogenolysis, thus converting the intracellular amino acids into the osmotically less active macromolecules [1]. Similarly, cell shrinkage stimulates and cell swelling inhibits glycogen degradation [1].

Cell volume further influences glucose and amino acid metabolism [1]. Cell swelling decreases glycolysis, increases flux through the pentose phosphate pathway, enhances lipogenesis from glucose, and inhibits transcription of phosphoenolpyruvate carboxykinase, a key enzyme for gluconeogenesis. Cell swelling stimulates oxidation of glycine and alanine, degradation of glutamine as well as generation of NH_4^+ and urea from amino acids. Cell swelling increases ketoisocaproate oxidation, acetyl CoA carboxylase and lipogenesis, decreases carnitine palmitoyltransferase I activity , lowers cytosolic ATP and phosphocreatine concentrations, enhances respiration and fosters RNA and DNA synthesis. Cell shrinkage exerts opposite metabolic effects.

The increased flux through the pentose phosphate pathway following cell swelling enhances NADPH production and thus increases the formation of glutathione (GSH). Conversely, NADPH production and GSH formation are decreased by cell shrinkage. Cell swelling thus increases, and cell shrinkage decreases cellular resistance to oxidative stress [1]. By the same token, cell shrinkage decreases the activity of NADPH oxidase and thus impedes cellular O_2^- formation. Thus, cell swelling increases and cell shrinkage decreases the formation of reactive oxygen species [1, 14].

The volume sensitivity of metabolism is exploited by hormones. Insulin swells liver cells by activation of both Na^+/H^+ exchange and Na^+, K^+, $2Cl^-$ cotransport and glucagon shrinks hepatocytes, presumably by activation of ion channels [14]. Insulin-induced cell swelling accounts for the antiproteolytic effect of the hormone and glucagon induced cell shrinkage accounts for the proteolytic effect of that hormone. Growth factors increase cell volume by stimulation of Na^+/H^+ exchange and partially of Na^+, K^+, $2Cl^-$ cotransport, an effect required for the stimulation of cell proliferation [5]. Along those lines, osmolyte flux is in the brain regulated by transmitters [15]. Given the impact of cell volume in hormonal action, the sensitivity of target cells to hormonal influence is expected to be influenced by alterations of cell volume.

Cell Volume-Sensitive Genes

Cell volume modifies the expression of a wide variety of genes [8, 16]. Altered gene expression may serve to adjust cellular osmolarity. For instance, cell shrinkage stimulates the expression of the Na^+, K^+, $2Cl^-$ cotransporter, the Na^+/K^+-ATPase α_1-subunit and enzymes or transporters engaged in cellular formation or accumulation of osmolytes including the aldose reductase as well as the Na^+-coupled transporters for betaine (BGT), taurine (NCT), myoinositol (SMIT) and amino acids. Other cell volume-sensitive genes encode proteins involved in the signaling of cell volume regulation. For instance, cell swelling stimulates the expression of the extracellular signal-regulated kinases ERK1, ERK2 and the Jun kinase-1, and cell shrinkage enhances the expression of the serum and glucocorticoid-inducible kinase SGK1 and cycloxygenase-2 [4, 8, 16, 17]. Other proteins are expressed to protect cells against excessive osmolarity [1]. For instance, cell shrinkage stimulates the expression of protein-stabilizing heat shock proteins [1]. Cell shrinkage stimulates expression and release of antidiuretic hormone ADH, a hormone retaining water and thus counteracting dehydration [1].

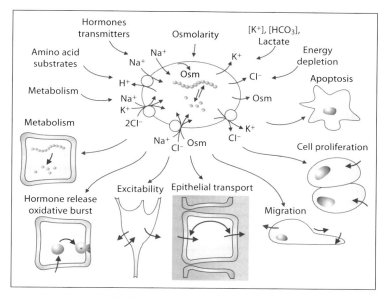

Fig. 2. Challenges of cell volume constancy and cell volume-sensitive functions.

Several cell volume-sensitive genes are seemingly unrelated to cell volume regulation [1]. For instance cell swelling stimulates the expression of β-actin and tubulin, of the immediate early genes c-jun and c-fos and the enzyme ornithine decarboxylase. Conversely, cell shrinkage stimulates the expression of the cytokine TNF-α, the Cl^- channel ClC-K1, P-glycoprotein, the immediate early genes Egr-1 and c-fos, the GTPase inhibitor $α_1$-chimaerin, the CDβ antigen, the enzymes phosphoenolpyruvate carboxykinase, arginine succinate lyase, tyrosine aminotransferase, tyrosine hydroxylase, dopamine β-hydroxylase, matrix metalloproteinase-9 and tissue plasminogen activator, as well as matrix proteins including biglycan and laminin B_2.

The stimulation of transcription is in part mediated by respective promoter regions in the cell volume-sensitive genes. Expression of the genes encoding aldose reductase, BGT and SGK1 are governed by osmolarity-responsive, tonicity-responsive (TonE) or cell volume-responsive elements. TonE binds the transcription factor TonE-binding protein, which is activated by cell shrinkage [16].

Signaling of Cell Volume Regulation

Sensors of cell volume and hydration remained elusive. Some evidence points to cellular protein content or macromolecular crowding [1]. The protein density may influence a serine/threonine kinase (see below), which in turn regulates the activity of cell volume regulatory KCl and Na$^+$, K$^+$, 2Cl$^-$ cotransport by respective phosphorylation of the transport proteins [4]. Alternatively, the cell could sense ionic strength or the concentration of individual ions such as Cl$^-$ [4], stretch on the cytoskeleton and/or cell membrane [4], change of the cell membrane curvature as well as activation of cytokine, Ca^{2+}-sensing receptors [18] and/or integrins [4].

The sensors stimulate a myriad of cellular signaling pathways, depending on cell type and functional state of a given cell [4]. In many cells, swelling increases intracellular activity of Ca^{2+}, which may enter through nonselective Ca^{2+} channels, Ca^{2+}-permeable members of the TRP (transient receptor potential) channel family, such as TRPV4, and L-type voltage-gated Ca^{2+} channels [4]. Ca^{2+} subsequently activates volume-regulatory K$^+$ channels and Cl$^-$ channels and influences other cell volume-sensitive cellular functions [4].

Cell volume affects cytoskeletal architecture and expression of cytoskeletal proteins [19]. Microtubules and actin filaments may participate in cell volume regulation, and their disruption may interfere with cell volume regulation. Alterations of cell volume modify the phosphorylation of a variety of proteins [4, 20]. Kinases activated during cell swelling include tyrosine kinases, protein kinase C, adenylate cyclase, MAP kinases, focal adhesion kinase (p121^{FAK}), phosphoinositide 3 (PI3) kinase and extracellular signal-regulated kinases ERK-1 and ERK-2 [4, 20]. Activation of PI3 kinase is followed by stimulation of protein kinase B (Akt) and the serum and glucocorticoid-inducible kinases which modify a wide variety of carriers and channels [17]. Expression of SGK1 is, however, downregulated by cell shrinkage, which disrupts SGK1-dependent signaling [17].

Osmotic cell shrinkage stimulates WNK (with no lysine kinase) 1 and 4, which in turn activate Ste-20-related proline alanine-rich kinase (SPAK) and oxidative stress-responsive kinase (OSR1) [21, 22]. SPAK and OSR1 activate the Na$^+$, K$^+$, 2Cl$^-$ cotransporters NKCC1 and NKCC2 [23]. Conversely, WNK4 inhibits KCl cotransporters [4]. WNK1 activates SGK1, which in turn inhibits WNK4 [4, 24]. Osmotic cell shrinkage further activates the tyrosine kinase Fyn, several MAP (mitogen-activated protein) kinase cascades, SAPK, p38 kinase, myosin light-chain kinase, Jun kinase, p21-activated kinases PAKs Rho kinase, LIM kinase and casein kinase [4, 20]. The kinases may influence cell volume regulation by modulating cytoskeleton, cell volume regulatory ion transport or activation of transcription factors governing expression of cell volume-regulated genes.

In some cells, swelling activates phospholipase A$_2$ resulting in the formation of the 15-lipoxygenase product hepoxilin A$_3$ and the 5-lipoxygenase product leukotriene LTD$_4$ [4]. The eicosanoids in turn stimulate cell volume-regulatory K$^+$ and/or Cl$^-$ channels and/or taurine release. Cell shrinkage may stimulate formation of PGE$_2$, which in turn may activate PGE$_2$-sensitive Na$^+$ channels [25]. Cell volume signaling may further involve nitric oxide [4, 26].

Cell swelling decreases and cell shrinkage increases the formation of phosphatidylinositol 4,5 bisphosphate [PtdIns(4,5)P$_2$] [4] by influencing the phosphatidylinositol 4-phosphate 5-kinase-β isoform (PIP5KIβ) [4]. PtdIns(4,5)P$_2$ stimulate some channels (TRPV1, ENaC), Na$^+$/H$^+$ exchange (NHE1) and Na$^+$/Ca^{2+} exchange and they inhibit TRPC6 [4, 27]. PtdIns(4,5)P$_2$ further stimulates actin polymerization [4, 28].

Cell swelling increases and cell shrinkage decreases the pH in acidic cellular compartments, including endosomes, lysosomes and secretory granules. The alkalinization of the acidic cellular compartments decreases protease activity and thus autophagic proteolysis [1]. By this means, cell swelling inhibits autophagic proteolysis [1].

Influence of Metabolism on Cell Volume

Cellular degradation of proteins to amino acids, glycogen to glucose phosphate, or triglycerides to glycerol and fatty acids results in an increased number of osmotically active particles, increased cellular osmolarity, and thus cell swelling. The degradation of the substrates to CO_2 and H_2O decreases cellular osmolarity and thus fosters cell shrinkage [1]. Glycolysis fosters cell swelling by cellular accumulation of lactate and H$^+$ and subsequent activation of the Na$^+$/H$^+$ exchanger [1].

Metabolic pathways may influence cell volume indirectly through alteration of transport across the cell membrane. In some cells, a decrease in cellular ATP could activate ATP-sensitive K$^+$ channels and thus lead to cell shrinkage. Formation of reactive oxygen species may shrink cells by activation of oxidant sensitive K$^+$ channels or by inhibition of oxidant sensitive Na$^+$, K$^+$, 2Cl$^-$ cotransport. By the same token, it could swell cells by inhibiting Kv1.3 K$^+$ channels and KCNE1/KCNQ1 K$^+$ channels [1].

In liver insufficiency, impaired formation of urea leads to accumulation of NH$_3$, which enters the brain, is taken up by glial cells, stimulates cellular formation and accumulation of glutamine and thus triggers glial cell swelling. Glial cells release myoinositol to counteract swelling and exhaustion of the osmolyte is followed by severe dysfunction leading to development of hepatic encephalopathy [14, 29].

In diabetic ketoacidosis, cell swelling may result from cellular accumulation of organic acids and cellular acidity activating the Na$^+$/H$^+$ exchanger as well as from hyperglycemia stimulating cellular formation and accumulation of sorbitol from glucose through aldose reductase [1]. Hyperglycemia further leads to formation of advanced glycation end products which upregulate SGK1 and similarly induce cell swelling [17]. To counteract cell swelling, cells release osmolytes such as myoinositol. Cell swelling inhibits proteolysis, fostering together with SGK1 the disposal of matrix proteins [30].

Hypercatabolic states, such as burns, acute pancreatitis, severe injury, or liver carcinoma may be caused by a decrease in muscle cell volume, which correlates with urea excretion, an indicator of protein degradation [1]. Conversely, hyper-catabolism can be reversed by glutamine, which swells cells by Na^+-coupled cellular uptake.

Cell Volume and Athletic Performance

A goal of exercise training is to produce cellular adaptations that, in turn, improve athletic performance. Given the considerable evidence from in vitro studies that cell shrinkage or swelling induces gene transcription and can impact carbohydrate and protein metabolism, it seems plausible to use hydration as a tool to manipulate cell signaling. There is supportive evidence, in vivo, that cell swelling can affect cell metabolism. For example, Keller et al. [31] reported that expansion of total body water (and induction of hyponatremia) produced modest reductions in resting protein breakdown (–6%) and protein catabolism (–20%) – observations consistent with in vitro cell swelling experiments.

The induction of overhydration also had effects on glucose and fat metabolism, as glucose disposal was reduced and glycerol appearance increased during an euglycemic hyperinsulinemic clamp. Together, the in vitro and in vivo observations suggest that manipulation of cellular hydration state might be a tool to promote favorable cellular adaptations.

Specific strategies exploiting cellular hydration to augment training adaptations, however, have not been established. A challenge in vivo is producing cell swelling and downstream metabolic signaling; water intake does not equate to cell swelling. The in vivo setting is also much more complex than in vitro, as hormones, cytokines, oxidative stress, etc. can potentially complicate the cellular metabolic responses to cell swelling and cell shrinkage. Strategies that exploit the effects of substances such as glutamine on cell volume may be more effective than simple manipulation of drinking behavior.

There is little doubt that glutamine decreases catabolism in vivo, and as shown in in vitro experiments, the antiproteolytic effect of glutamine is completely lost if glutamine-induced cell swelling is prevented. The experiments conducted to date have been focused on furthering our understanding of the physiological consequences of cell swelling and shrinkage, and the mechanisms responsible for these effects. Very little research has been done to date to examine if cell swelling can be exploited to facilitate exercise training.

Conclusions

Cells are equipped with cell volume-regulatory mechanisms adjusting cell volume to the functional demands. The mechanisms are under the control of diverse signaling pathways. Conversely, cell volume and cell volume-sensitive cellular functions participate in a wide variety of physiological and pathophysiological mechanisms including regulation of metabolism. Understanding the interplay of cell volume and metabolic regulation may open novel opportunities for favorably influencing several clinical disorders such as diabetes, renal or hepatic insufficiency, catabolic states and fibrosing disease. Strategies that exploit cell volume regulation may also have applications in exercise training adaptation.

References

1 Lang F, Busch GL, Ritter M, et al: Functional significance of cell volume regulatory mechanisms. Physiol Rev 1998;78:247–306.
2 King LS, Kozono D, Agre P: From structure to disease: the evolving tale of aquaporin biology. Nat Rev Mol Cell Biol 2004;5: 687–698.
3 Haussinger D: Osmosensing and osmosignaling in the liver. Wien Med Wochenschr 2008;158:549–552.
4 Hoffmann EK, Lambert IH, Pedersen SF: Physiology of cell volume regulation in vertebrates. Physiol Rev 2009;89:193–277.
5 Lang F, Foller M, Lang K, et al: Cell volume regulatory ion channels in cell proliferation and cell death. Methods Enzymol 2007;428: 209–225.
6 Pasantes-Morales H, Cruz-Rangel S: Brain volume regulation: osmolytes and aquaporin perspectives. Neuroscience 2010;168: 871–884.
7 Usher-Smith JA, Huang CL, Fraser JA: Control of cell volume in skeletal muscle. Biol Rev Camb Philos Soc 2009;84:143–159.
8 Burg MB, Ferraris JD, Dmitrieva NI: Cellular response to hyperosmotic stresses. Physiol Rev 2007;87:1441–1474.
9 Beck FX, Neuhofer W: Cell volume regulation in the renal papilla. Contrib Nephrol 2006;152:181–197.
10 Wehner F: Cell volume-regulated cation channels. Contrib Nephrol 2006;152:25–53.
11 Okada Y: Cell volume-sensitive chloride channels: phenotypic properties and molecular identity. Contrib Nephrol 2006;152:9–24.
12 Jakab M, Grundbichler M, Benicky J, et al: Glucose induces anion conductance and cytosol-to-membrane transposition of ICln in INS-1E rat insulinoma cells. Cell Physiol Biochem 2006;18:21–34.
13 Wehner F, Olsen H, Tinel H, et al: Cell volume regulation: osmolytes, osmolyte transport, and signal transduction. Rev Physiol Biochem Pharmacol 2003;148:1–80.
14 Haussinger D, Gorg B: Interaction of oxidative stress, astrocyte swelling and cerebral ammonia toxicity. Curr Opin Clin Nutr Metab Care 2010;13:87–92.
15 Fisher SK, Heacock AM, Keep RF, et al: Receptor regulation of osmolyte homeostasis in neural cells. J Physiol 2010;588: 3355–3364.
16 Ferraris JD, Burg MB: Tonicity-dependent regulation of osmoprotective genes in mammalian cells; in Lang F (ed): Mechanisms and Significance of Cell Volume Regulation. Contrib Nephrol. Basel, Karger, 2006, vol 152, pp 125–141.
17 Lang F, Bohmer C, Palmada M, et al: (Patho)physiological significance of the serum- and glucocorticoid-inducible kinase isoforms. Physiol Rev 2006;86:1151–1178.
18 Fiol DF, Kultz D: Osmotic stress sensing and signaling in fishes. FEBS J 2007;274: 5790–5798.
19 Tamma G, Procino G, Strafino A, et al: Hypotonicity induces aquaporin-2 internalization and cytosol-to-membrane translocation of ICln in renal cells. Endocrinology 2007;148:1118–1130.
20 Schliess F, Haussinger D: Osmosensing and signaling in the regulation of liver function. Contrib Nephrol 2006;152:198–209.
21 Delpire E, Austin TM: Kinase regulation of Na-K-2Cl cotransport in primary afferent neurones. J Physiol, Epub ahead of print.
22 Zagorska A, Pozo-Guisado E, Boudeau J, et al: Regulation of activity and localization of the WNK1 protein kinase by hyperosmotic stress. J Cell Biol 2007;176:89–100.

23 Delpire E, Gagnon KB: SPAK and OSR1:STE20 kinases involved in the regulation of ion homoeostasis and volume control in mammalian cells. Biochem J 2008;409:321–331.

24 Peng JB, Warnock DG: WNK4-mediated regulation of renal ion transport proteins. Am J Physiol Renal Physiol 2007;293:F961–F973.

25 Lang PA, Kasinathan RS, Brand VB, et al: Accelerated clearance of plasmodium-infected erythrocytes in sickle cell trait and annexin-A7 deficiency. Cell Physiol Biochem 2009;24:415–428.

26 Kucherenko Y, Browning J, Tattersall A, et al: Effect of peroxynitrite on passive K+ transport in human red blood cells. Cell Physiol Biochem 2005; 15:271–280.

27 Gamper N, Shapiro MS: Target-specific PIP(2) signalling: how might it work? J Physiol 2007;582:967–975.

28 Janmey PA, Lindberg U: Cytoskeletal regulation: rich in lipids. Nat Rev Mol Cell Biol 2004;5:658–666.

29 Heins J, Zwingmann C: Organic osmolytes in hyponatremia and ammonia toxicity. Metab Brain Dis 2010;25:81–89.

30 Feng Y, Wang Q, Wang Y, et al: SGK1-mediated fibronectin formation in diabetic nephropathy. Cell Physiol Biochem 2005;16:237–244.

31 Keller U, Szinnai G, Bilz S, Berneis K: Effects of changes in hydration on protein, glucose and lipid metabolism in man: impact on health. Eur J Clin Nutr 2003;57(suppl 2):569–574.

Discussion

Dr. Montain: Your observations that cell volume can alter cell metabolism leads to the idea that manipulating hydration to produce swelling or shrinking could be a tool to promote adaptation. In your in vitro model, are the cells responsive to osmotic challenges in the 270–300 mosm range? How much 'slop' does the cell accommodate before a response is produced?

Dr. Lang: That's a very good question. As you may have seen, only a few percent of cell volume changes are required to modify cell function. The effect of insulin on cell volume is only 8% cell swelling. That extent of cell swelling is sufficient to stop proteolysis. I should add that effects of insulin are not exclusively cell volume mediated, and there is extensive signaling of insulin which is not directly related to cell volume but is only modified by alterations of cell volume. The effect of insulin on proteolysis, however, is almost completely due to cell swelling. The sensitivity of cells to alterations of cell volume is exquisite, and only a 1% change of cell volume may activate channels and transporters.

Dr. Montain: So, the cell is responsive to an osmolarity step change between 280–290, 280–300 mosm?

Dr. Lang: If you force the cell to swell by reducing extracellular osmolarity, it regulates its volume rapidly and the cell swelling is only transient. Frequently, the cells do not regulate completely and thus, a residual change of cell volume persists. If you add glutamine, you observe sustained cell swelling. Under those conditions, volume regulation prevents further increase in cell volume but, in that case, some 4% cell swelling is maintained, which is not necessarily true if you change osmolarity. Similarly, if you add insulin or any other hormone which upregulates cell volume, then you observe a sustained effect.

Dr. Montain: Often, in the cell culture experiments, a step change of a fairly large magnitude is applied. Do you see different cell responses if the stress is smaller and applied in a graded manner?

Dr. Lang: There is the so called isovolumetric cell volume regulation: If you change osmolarity very slowly, then the cell may not swell or shrink appreciably, because it regulates fast enough to avoid cell volume changes to the extent that we can measure it. The cells are better in measuring their volume than we are, so our methods are only able to pick the cell volume changes when the cell is already stimulated extensively. Accordingly, upon very slow osmolarity change, you do not see any changes in cell volume, yet you stimulate cell volume regulation.

Dr. Zemel: Can you comment on the consequences of cell volume changes that are iso-osmotic, for example cell volume changes consequent to increases or decreases in fat droplet size – how might this impact SGK1? Also, what about the tissue distribution of SGK1?

Dr. Lang: For many years, I have wondered whether or not fat droplets in a cell are relevant for cell volume. I do not believe they are, but I have no data to show that. The belief is based on the consideration that the protein concentration does not change when you accumulate triglycerides in the cell, and to the extent that cell volume regulatory mechanisms are triggered by alterations of the cytosolic protein concentration, addition of triglycerides would not stimulate cell volume regulation. However, this is mere speculation.

Dr. Haschke: What is the effect on the cell if somebody is treated with IGF-I, which stimulates insulin secretion? Is there a visible effect, and if so, does this explain the symptom of headache observed during treatment?

Dr. Lang: IGF-I stimulates SGK1, which in turn stimulates sodium potassium cotransport. This leads to cell swelling; that is to say, IGF-I may lead to cell swelling. Whether or not that occurs in glial cells and in neurons to the extent that intracerebral pressure increases, I don't know, but that's an interesting comment.

Dr. Spriet: My question relates to skeletal muscle, particularly during exercise. I noticed that you presented one slide from a patient population where you appear to have an estimate of cell water in muscle. Do you have any information on the impact of whole-body dehydration on skeletal muscle? In other words, how well defended is the cell volume of active skeletal muscle during exercise?

Dr. Lang: The skeletal muscle volume measurements I showed were the work of Dr. Roth in Vienna. He calculated the intracellular water content from the chloride concentration. We do not have data during exercise or dehydration.

Dr. Maughan: Many years ago, we did some studies on the osmotic fragility of the red blood cell because you can easily incubate them and measure cell swelling as osmolarity is manipulated. Some of the cells were much more sensitive to changes in osmotic pressure than others because they didn't all burst at the same osmolarity, and exercise seemed to increase the osmotic fragility of the red cells. What is it that exercise is doing to the cell that is changing its ability to tolerate that swelling?

Dr. Lang: We have no experience with cell volume regulation of erythrocytes following exercise. However, there is a powerful machinery linking volume and survival of erythrocytes. Similar to nucleated cells, erythrocytes undergo suicidal death upon excessive cell shrinkage, a phenomenon called eryptosis. They express a cation channel, which is calcium permeable. If you shrink them, they open that cation channel leading to increases in cytosolic calcium, calcium-sensitive scrambling of the cell membrane, and phosphatidylserine exposure on the cell surface. Phosphatidylserine-exposing erythrocytes are eventually removed. This mechanism is important for the removal of injured cells.

Dr. Maughan: We certainly saw a big increase in the osmotic fragility after a marathon race – so that's a very acute effect on the cells. A second question: you say there are no cells with a significant hydrostatic pressure, but in the situation of hyponatremic encephalopathy where individuals drink so much that plasma sodium concentration falls, the brain swells, and there is increased intracranial pressure that may lead to circulatory occlusion. Why isn't there a regulatory mechanism that overrides the osmotic effect and prevents the increase in pressure?

Dr. Lang: It usually works very well; otherwise, we would face this problem all the time. Of course, the single glial cell which regulates its volume doesn't think about the circulation and about the pressure. The small increase in pressure, sufficient to stop cerebral perfusion, is negligible as compared to osmotic pressure gradients. Accordingly, you cannot squeeze out neuronal cells by increasing intracerebral pressure. There is another problem: during cerebral cell volume regulation, cellular potassium is not released into the blood, but rather into the cerebral interstitial fluid, where it leads to local increases in extracellular potassium concentration. As a result, the brain is not very well able to maintain osmotic equilibrium, making it extremely important for the brain to be bathed in an isotonic environment. Cerebral cells regulate their volume mainly utilizing organic osmolytes, a mechanism which is very slow.

Dr. Baar: With regard to insulin and swelling effects, how much is dependent on stretch-activated channels rather than some indirect effect of opening or closing of channels?

Dr. Lang: The stretch-activated channels are the last line of defense. They usually are not important for daily life, and not for insulin effects. Nevertheless, the stretch-activated channels were the first discovered direct mechanism of cell volume regulation. Thus, the scientific community was very excited about those channels. ADH-releasing cells express stretch-inactivated channels, so that when the stretch reduces they are activated. But otherwise, the mechanosensitive channels are not so important for cell volume regulation and they are not involved in the effects of insulin.

Dr. Phillips: In clinical situations like burns and sepsis, treating the patients with osmolytic solutions containing glutamine as well as other substances, produces positive outcomes. In the sports supplement market, people have tried to exploit these data using osmolytic compounds like glutamine, taurine and creatine for example, but normal skeletal muscle doesn't seem very responsive. In your cell culture model, do these approaches affect protein synthesis or protein breakdown such that the cells appear to be in a better state?

Dr. Lang: This is a very interesting question. We almost failed to see the insulin effect by looking at resistant cells. When Dieter tried the effect of insulin in fed rats, he did not see anything. Only when he took livers of starved rats, did he discover the effect of insulin. Obviously, you need prior shrinkage to see the effect of insulin. We now know that SGK1, which is required for the full effect of insulin on cell volume, is a cell volume-regulated gene which is downregulated in a swollen cell. To see a full effect of insulin, SGK1 must be expressed. Along those lines, possibly only a dehydrated skeletal muscle expresses high levels of SGK1. That is just a speculation at the moment. As long as SGK1 is high, the swelling effect is apparent. If SGK1 is low, no effect is observed. Possibly the resting normal skeletal muscle does not respond because it has very low SGK1 levels. Again, we need to do the measurements to test whether this explanation is correct.

Dr. Phillips: Is it fair to conclude that so called osmolytic substances like creatine or taurine have limited effect in normal skeletal muscle?

Dr. Lang: The effect of creatine would depend on how much creatine transporter is expressed and that depends on how much SGK1 is expressed. So, I think it's not as simple that you consume the substances, then the cells take up the substance and swell. You may need to go further upstream in the signaling pathway to modify taurine uptake or creatine uptake in a skeletal muscle which is not shrunken.

Dr. van Loon: With exercise, there are massive changes in osmolarity in the muscle cell. The increase in cell volume will trigger cell volume regulation mechanisms, but may also stimulate metabolism. Based on your observations, do you think these changes in osmolarity lead to changes in the myonuclear domain and therefore contribute to muscle hypertrophy?

Dr. Lang: Osmolarity changes metabolism and metabolism may, of course, change the cell volume. Signaling is not a chain of events, but a network with mutual interactions. If you fully understand the system, then you can exploit that knowledge to manipulate cell volume and metabolism. However, you should not expect a simple means to elicit the desired effect. The underlying mechanisms are of course regulated by negative feedback, which adds complexity to the mutual interaction between osmolarity changes and metabolism.

Dr. van Loon: Is an increase in cell volume following exercise a setoff point for cell activation and ultimately greater myonuclear content and muscle hypertrophy?

Dr. Lang: I think if you swell a cell, you set the stage for net protein synthesis. The lipid metabolism is less sensitive to cell volume. The most sensitive metabolic pathway is certainly proteolysis and the second is glycogenolysis.

Dr. van Loon: So, if you design an experiment to pharmaceutically prevent rehydration or cell volume increase following exercise you would prevent the adaptive response to exercise? Is it so crucial?

Dr. Lang: The experiment has yet to be done, but my expectation would be yes, it has a major impact. Please remember that 8% of cell volume change is the full effect of insulin on proteolysis in the liver. Cell swelling is really a highly effective, very powerful mechanism regulating metabolism. We have not done the experiment with skeletal muscle, but my prediction would be you won't be able to produce net protein synthesis if you don't allow the cell to reswell and to overcome cell shrinkage.

Dr. Maughan: To follow on from this point, we have recently done a pilot study in which every other day during an 8-week training period, subjects ingested sufficient glycerol to drive up plasma glycerol concentrations by ~20 mm. Presumably, this glycerol dosing would cause a transient cellular dehydration. We don't have any muscle tissues to examine if the stimulus affected skeletal muscle signaling, but there has been no benefit in terms of muscle strength or muscle size.

Dr. Lang: I recommend an experiment determining whether or not exercise would have an effect in the SGK1 knockout mice or not. My expectation is that exercise will upregulate SGK1, and the SGK1 will enhance cell swelling, and the cell swelling sets the stage for more protein synthesis and less protein degradation.

Dr. Baar: Just to follow on from that, we have seen using downstream targets of SGK1 that mTOR seems to be an important part of SGK1 activation.

Dr. Lang: You are perfectly right, and the effect of mTOR for instance on creatine transporter depends on SGK1.

Dr. Baar: Can you comment on your preliminary studies of the physical activity of SGK1 knockout mice?

Dr. Lang: Yes, they run at the same speed but they become exhausted more rapidly. When we placed them on a running wheel, the knockout mice did not run as far as the wild type mice under otherwise identical conditions. But, I think I would need an expert like you to perform the respective experiments in a really professional way.

Dr. McLaughlin: A lot of the plasma membrane-mediated signaling events and channel activities are modulated by the composition of the plasma membrane and lipids in particular. Is there any evidence that the composition of the plasma membrane or altering the composition of the plasma membrane affects the cell response to volume regulation?

Dr. Lang: Yes, that has been done by others. Cell volume regulation is for instance influenced by cholesterol content of the plasma membrane. We have never done these types of experiments, so I can't say much more.

Dr. Baar: We are going to talk later about how you might try to accelerate a stress beforehand, for example by manipulating glycogen content, and how that can augment the adaptations that occur with exercise. Would there be any merit to an approach where you try to dehydrate prior to resistance exercise to sort of prime the protein synthesis response and then following the resistance exercise training, restore fluid and provide the amino acids?

Dr. Lang: I would go another way. Again you are the experts in skeletal muscle, I am just expert in SGK1 and in cell volume regulation, you have to do the experiments, but I would try to upregulate SGK1 without shrinkage. The shrinkage would be counterproductive. I would try to upregulate SGK1 and then add a stimulus for SGK1, and then you would get dramatic swelling and would have hopefully dramatic protein synthesis and inhibition of protein degradation. There are several means to stimulate SGK1 without shrinking the cells. SGK1 is regulated in two steps, first there is genomic regulation which is required for the activation, and then there is activation. Insulin is only activating, so if there is no SGK1 around, insulin cannot activate it.

Dr. Baar: I wonder if cell swelling isn't one of the mechanisms underlying the occlusion growth paradigm, where hypertrophy is induced by inflating a cuff to cut off blood flow during low-intensity exercise. This approach produces a period of osmotic stress which magnifies a very small exercise stimulus with a huge blood flow stimulus.

Dr. Lang: Ischemia is one of the mechanisms upregulating SGK1 expression, so that could be one practical way to do what I just suggested.

Dr. Montain: In your studies, have you examined whether there is adaptation to a repeated stimulus? Do the cells need a greater challenge to produce a response or do the cells basically have a very short memory so a pulsatile challenge repeatedly produces the same cellular activation?

Dr. Lang: We have not exactly done that experiment. When you shrink the cells continuously, then you have a sustained increase in SGK1 expression. Likewise, if you stimulate the cell with TGF-β, you have a sustained increase in SGK1 expression. However, if you stimulate expression with interleukin-4, then you have only a transient increase in SGK1 expression. So, whether SGK1 is upregulated transiently or in a sustained manner seems to depend on the stimulus.

Concluding Comments

Maughan RJ, Burke LM (eds): Sports Nutrition: More Than Just Calories – Triggers for Adaptation.
Nestlé Nutr Inst Workshop Ser, vol 69, pp 131–149,
Nestec Ltd., Vevey/S. Karger AG., Basel, © 2011

Practical Nutritional Recommendations for the Athlete

Ronald J. Maughan[a] · Louise M. Burke[b]

[a]Loughborough University, Loughborough, UK; [b]Sports Nutrition, Australian Institute of Sport,
Canberra, ACT, Australia

Abstract

The aim of training is to achieve optimum performance on the day of competition via
three processes or paradigms; training hard to create the required training stimulus, training smart to maximize adaptations to the training stimulus, and training specifically to
fine-turn the behaviors or physiology needed for competition strategies. Dietary strategies for competition must target the factors that would otherwise cause fatigue during
the event, promoting an enhancement of performance by reducing or delaying the onset
of these factors. In some cases, the nutritional strategies needed to achieve these various
paradigms are different, and even opposite to each other, so athletes need to periodize
their nutrition, just as they periodize their training program. The evolution of new knowledge from sports nutrition research, such as presented in this book, usually starts with a
stark concept that must be further refined; to move from individual nutrients to food,
from 'one size fits all' to the individual needs and practices of different athletes, and from
single issues to an integrated picture of sports nutrition. The translation from science to
practice usually requires a large body of follow-up studies as well as experimentation in
the field.

Introduction

The origins of sports nutrition date back as far back as the earliest records of
sporting competition: the original Olympians in Greece believed that certain
foods would confer strength or other special attributes to assist performance.
However, the science of sports nutrition really gained momentum only in
the 1960s when Scandinavian sports scientists used the percutaneous biopsy
technique to examine muscle substrates, muscle enzymes and the capacity for
exercise. They found that, by altering dietary intake in extreme ways, recent

nutrition influenced fuel use and cycling endurance. A half-century later we are still refining the practical details of the technique known as carbohydrate loading that emanated from their work. This episode demonstrates the general way in which sports nutrition has evolved. Typically, some scientific technique is undertaken to measure the effects of a dietary manipulation and a gross result is reported. While this may receive much attention in scientific journals, it needs further refinement and filtering before it is fully translated into optimum practice in the real-life world of sport.

This book has provided a series of reviews of topics that are cutting edge in sports science; the aim of this final chapter is to summarize the ways in which the current knowledge in these areas can be implemented into athletic practice and to highlight some of the limitations and potential pitfalls. Before undertaking this, however, it is worth considering the principles of training to understand how the interaction of exercise and nutrition can adapt the body to enhance its function. It is also important to consider the challenges of translating science into practice.

An Overview of the Principles of Training

The aim of athletic training is to enhance performance by altering the various physiological, mechanical, metabolic, psychological and other factors that limit exercise performance. The basic principles of athletic training are well established. A well-designed program based on the principle of progressive overload should result in an improvement in performance that is proportional to the training stimulus. The training load can be quantified in terms of the intensity, duration and frequency of the individual training sessions. Training may last no more than a few minutes on one or two days per week for the child or novice athlete or for the athlete returning from injury, but elite athletes in most sports will undertake one or more training sessions per day, each lasting an hour or longer. Within limits, increasing the training load will result in greater improvements in performance. There are limits, however, and overtraining will have negative effects on both health and performance.

Training is more than simply undertaking the athlete's specific event or sport. Most athletes undertake a variety of training modes or practices that target the muscle or whole body characteristics that will achieve enhancements of performance. Such training is highly specific: muscles that are not trained will not adapt and the changes taking place in the structural and functional properties of the muscles are specific to the nature of the training stimulus [1]. Strength training should increase muscle strength, but will have little effect on endurance capacity. Endurance training, on the other hand, has little or no effect on muscle strength – marathon runners generally have a small muscle mass and low muscle strength in spite of very high volumes of training. To achieve these adaptations, the muscle must respond with a selective stimulation of muscle protein synthesis and degradation: the aim is to make more of the proteins that promote performance while breaking down some of those proteins that do not contribute to performance. These adaptations must occur not only in skeletal muscle but in all other tissues that influence performance.

At one time, it was thought that the primary role of sports nutrition was to support consistent intensive training by allowing the athlete to train harder without succumbing to illness, injury and chronic fatigue. It is increasingly recognized, however, that nutrition interventions can allow athletes to train 'smarter' rather than just training harder. This can allow athletes to maximize the adaptations taking place in muscle and other tissues without risking over-training. In sports where skill and tactics are major elements in successful performance, good nutrition strategies might allow the same level of fitness to be achieved with less training, allowing more time to be devoted to technical work while also reducing the risk of chronic fatigue and injury.

A final role of training is to prepare the athlete to undertake the nutritional strategies that will be important in their competition eating plan. Although training prepares the athlete to get to the starting line or opening phase of their event, performance can be further fine-tuned by nutritional practices undertaken before, during or after (between) competition bouts. These practices must specifically target nutritionally influenced factors that limit performance, such as depletion of fuel stores or disturbances to homeostasis. Competition nutrition strategies may include the targeted intake of fluid and carbohydrate in the days and hours prior to the event, as well as fluid, carbohydrate, electrolytes and perhaps other nutrients during exercise. Where a series of bouts is required to determine the outcome of competition, the intake of carbohydrate, protein, fluid and electrolytes may be part of promoting recovery between events. Practicing competition strategies during the training phase, particularly the consumption of fluids and foods during exercise, is an important part of the preparation. Part of the process may be adapting the plan to the athlete, so that competition fluid and food intake is adjusted to suit individual tolerance and opportunities for nutrient intake during the event. However, there is also opportunity to adapt the athlete to the plan, to learn the behavioral skills associated with obtaining and consuming fluids and foods during exercise and to train the gut to tolerate or process the ingested nutrients.

Translating Sports Science Research to Practice in the Field

The scientific process typically starts with the testing of a hypothesis. To provide the best opportunity to see a measurable effect of the intervention under scrutiny, the initial studies are usually undertaken with a large dose or a lengthy duration of application. Typically, the intervention is presented as a single entity, under baseline metabolic conditions (e.g. fasted), which bears little resemblance to everyday nutrition or the conditions of sport. Sometimes, sophisticated methodologies are available: the use of percutaneous biopsies to measure characteristics of the muscle, the use of radioactive or stable isotope tracers to follow the utilization or storage of nutrients, or the use of magnetic resonance spectroscopy or other nuclear medicine techniques to measure changes in metabolites. However, the expense and logistics associated with these techniques have implications for the number and caliber of subjects in experiments.

There are many reasons to study the interaction of nutrition and exercise, with worthy outcomes aimed at prevention and treatment of community health issues such as diabetes, obesity or sarcopenia. Many studies do not therefore have a primary interest in sporting outcomes, or even the performance of exercise. Indeed, the measurement of sports performance is a highly challenging area, with most scientific investigations being unable to detect the changes or differences in performance that would be worthwhile in the world of competitive sport, where millimeters and milliseconds can separate the winners from the rest of the field [2]. In some of the newest research techniques, scientists can measure factors that underpin the function of an exercising muscle or the process of its adaptation to exercise (e.g. enzymes, signaling proteins, transcription factors). While these factors are critical in explaining the mechanisms of function or adaptation, they are often used as a proxy for exercise capacity, which becomes a proxy for sports performance per se. Enhanced access to scientific reports, via media such as PubMed or sports science websites and blogs, means that there is rapid communication of 'breakthrough' studies of nutrition and exercise interaction to sports scientists, coaches and athletes themselves. All these factors interact to create enthusiasm in the sports world for the results of diet-exercise studies, but they can also make it difficult to find a direct application of the results to the athlete.

In an ideal world, once a tested hypothesis provides information about a nutritional intervention that could be promising to the athlete or sports performance, further studies would take place to determine how the information can be applied to conditions of sport. This would include dose-response studies to delineate the ideal amount, timing and duration of an intervention, and the best opportunity to use it within an athlete's periodized program of training and competition. Suitable or ideal forms of the intervention might be tested, ranging from individual nutrients, special sports foods or supplements to everyday foods. It should be tested on athletes of different gender, age, training history and sporting caliber to identify the suitable recipient(s) of the intervention. The application to different sports, different events, and different individuals should also be investigated to account for the various factors that ultimately limit performance as well as the individuality of responses between athletes. Interactions with other interventions or practices in sport need to be considered, and ultimately, an appropriate measurement of performance should be tested to confirm the benefit. Even when all this is undertaken, the final analysis will require consideration of the practicality or logistics of the intervention: for example, can the athlete afford it (in expense or energy considerations)?; is it accessible and available (can it be found or undertaken within the athlete's environment or restraints)?; does it integrate with the athlete's other nutritional goals?; is it safe and ethical (are there side effects from its use; is it allowable within any anti-doping codes that exist)?

Understandably, this 'ideal world' is too intricate to be realistic. Therefore, the translation of most sports science research into practice relies mostly on interpolation and extrapolation of the available studies as well as individual experimentation in the field. In providing an analysis of the practical applications of the nutritional interventions reviewed in this book, we have had to undertake a theoretical cost-benefit analysis of the available information.

Role of Protein before, during and after Training

It is clear from studies that have measured rates of whole body or muscle-specific protein synthesis and breakdown that there is a transient increase in the rate of protein breakdown after an exercise bout [for review, see 3]. The intensity and duration of exercise necessary to trigger this effect either minimally or optimally are unknown, as the present dose-response studies are neither consistent in their findings nor exhaustive in their investigation. The coach and athlete know, however, that there is a threshold for the training stimulus below which adaptation will not occur. A single bout of intense resistance training will increase net protein synthesis for a period lasting from about 24 to 48 h [3]. For muscle hypertrophy to occur, net protein synthesis must exceed net protein breakdown, and muscle growth occurs through the cumulative effect of repeated periods of positive protein balance. However, it is often the case in sport that mature, already well-trained athletes do not seek to achieve muscle hypertrophy, as an increase in mass would bring a weight penalty that could impair performance. Similarly, the goal of endurance training is not to achieve a gain in muscle mass. Instead, a change in the muscle protein composition is sought by selective stimulation of synthesis and breakdown of specific proteins.

The available evidence suggests that it is the essential amino acids, and perhaps specifically leucine, that are effective in stimulating protein synthesis when ingested around the time of an exercise session [4, 5]. However, this should not be taken as an indication that ingestion of leucine itself, of a mixture of branched chain amino acids, or a mixture that includes all of the essential amino acids is necessarily the best strategy for athletes to adopt. Mixed protein sources that include both essential and non-essential amino acids may be just as effective as essential amino acids alone, and have advantages in terms of cost, convenience and palatability. These include animal protein sources such as meat, fish and

Table 1. Typical portion sizes for a variety of foods [52], food portion size that will provide 20 g of protein, total energy content [53], and total amounts of essential amino acids (EAA) and leucine in this food portion size [54]

Food	Typical portion size, g	Amount for 20 g protein, g	Energy content		Total EAA g	Leucine g
			kcal	kJ		
Bread (white)	75	238	559	2,385	6.48	1.48
Spaghetti (boiled)	50	667	574	2,435	10.11	2.20
Milk (semi-skimmed)	195	606	279	1,182	10.27	2.03
Egg (raw)	60	160	235	979	9.58	1.63
Steak, stewing (raw)	175	99	174	729	9.16	1.60
Chicken (roast, light meat)	85	75	106	449	8.52	1.49
Lentils (boiled)	155	263	263	1,115	7.91	1.55
Potato (new, boiled)	150	1,333	1,000	3,972	7.58	1.27

Note the very different amounts of food and the different energy contents for the same amount of total protein and for similar amounts of EAA.

seafood, poultry, eggs and many dairy foods (milk, cheese, yoghurt, etc.), as well as the complementing of plant-rich proteins (e.g. soy and grains; see table 1). Ultimately, the athlete wants to know the amount, the type and the timing of intake of protein sources over the day, and in relation to an exercise bout, that they should consume to achieve their desired adaptation to training. The interaction of the composition of the amino acids in these foods and their rate of digestion and release of amino acids into the blood may alter their final effect on muscle protein synthesis.

Moore et al. [6] examined the relationship between increasing amounts of protein (in the form of egg protein) ingestion and postexercise muscle protein synthesis. The fractional synthetic rate of mixed muscle protein increased with increasing amounts of protein intake until an amount of 20 g was consumed: this corresponds to an intake of about 9 g of essential amino acids. Doubling the dose to 40 g had little further effect on protein synthesis, so it seems reasonable to recommend an intake of about 20–25 g of high-quality protein after training. Subjects in this study had a mean body mass of 86 kg with a large individual variation in body size. All were given the same fixed amounts of protein without any adjustment for body mass, and there was apparently no suggestion that the dose should be adjusted for body size, but it might seem prudent when dealing with subjects at the extremes of body mass to adjust the protein dose

Maughan · Burke

accordingly. Table 1 shows the amounts of various protein foods that are necessary to provide 20 g of protein, and shows the essential amino acid content and leucine content of these foods: it also includes the total energy content of this food portion. Although various foods can provide the necessary amounts of protein and of essential amino acids, some foods would have to be eaten in improbably large amounts to achieve this, and would provide inappropriately large amounts of energy.

The present research suggests that the overall muscle protein synthetic response is influenced by the effect of dietary protein sources on plasma amino acid profiles. Whey protein seems most effective in stimulating muscle protein synthesis when ingested after exercise. This may be partly the result of its rapid digestion and absorption [7]. However, soy protein drinks cause a faster and more pronounced rise in plasma total amino acid concentration than occurs after ingestion of the same amount of protein in the form of milk proteins, but the milk results in a greater stimulation of protein synthesis and a greater net protein balance in the exercised muscle [8], perhaps as a result of its higher leucine content.

It is not feasible to undertake tracer studies to determine which dietary proteins achieve the highest rates of muscle protein synthesis. Indeed it is likely that the ingestion of a number and combination of different protein sources will be able, when combined with appropriate exercise, to achieve good results towards the athlete's goals. In addition to knowing the amount of protein and leucine in a protein-rich food source, a rating of the speed of digestion of this food and its effect of plasma amino acid concentrations (i.e. which protein sources are 'fast' and which are 'slow', when eaten alone or in combination with other foods) might help the athlete to choose foods to consume to provide the desired amino acid profile. There is not complete agreement on the preferred time to consume a protein source in relation to a bout of exercise per se, with some studies showing that intake before and during a session is of benefit, while others show that soon after exercise is optimal [for review, see 9]. Of course, whatever the desired time point for achieving a desired elevation of amino acid profiles, there may be an interaction of the timing, type and amount of proteins ingested to achieve this. For example, it may be possible to achieve the same amino acid concentration with a small amount of a 'fast' protein food which achieves a peak amino acid concentration after 30 min (such as whey or a liquid protein like milk) as by eating a larger amount of protein in the form of a 'slow' protein (casein or a solid meat meal) at a time point an hour earlier than this.

It should be noted that there is a time lag between the peak plasma amino acid response and the muscle protein synthetic response. Plasma amino acid concentrations peak about 30 min after ingestion of a fast protein source at the completion of a resistance exercise bout, with concentrations returning to the fasting baseline within about 3 h of ingestion; however, the muscle protein synthetic response appears to reach peak levels at 3–5 h [7]. Since the muscle protein synthetic response is increased above baseline for 24–48 h after a single resistance bout, the timing and amounts of protein consumed over the rest of the day also need to be considered. Repeated ingestion of small amounts of protein at frequent intervals may maximize net protein accretion. This accords with the reported practice of some bodybuilders who consume protein at intervals of no more than 2–3 h over the whole day, and bodybuilders are often recommended to eat protein at least 5–7 times per day during periods of training [10]. However, the muscle is also saturable after a single feeding of protein [6] and refractory to further intake of protein [11], so it is also possible that a more spread out pattern of protein intake might allow protein synthesis to be 'turned off' before it is then turned on maximally again. Studies of such hypotheses are required.

Athletes have been accustomed to ingestion of carbohydrate soon after training to begin the process of muscle glycogen resynthesis [12]. There have been some suggestions that addition of carbohydrate to protein ingested after exercise might further stimulate protein synthesis on account of the anabolic action of an elevated circulating insulin concentration. Borsheim et al. [13] showed an increased leg uptake of amino acids when carbohydrate was coingested with protein, suggesting an increased net protein synthesis. However, in a more recent study, even the ingestion of a very large amount of carbohydrate together with a large bolus of protein hydrolysate (0.3 g•kg^{-1}•h^{-1} protein hydrolysate with 0, 0.15, or 0.6 g•kg^{-1}•h^{-1} carbohydrate during a 6-hour recovery period) was not effective in promoting further increases in muscle protein synthesis [14].

Most of these studies have focused on the effects of various feeding strategies on acute measures of whole body or muscle protein synthesis, but the athlete's concern is with functional outcomes. Training studies to investigate the efficacy of feeding varying types and amounts of different proteins at varying times after different types of training are extremely complex and time-consuming, so it is not surprising that there are few experimental studies. It is perhaps more surprising that there are any at all. Hartman et al. [15] investigated the effects of feeding skimmed milk, soy or carbohydrate after training in young novice weightlifters. Subjects trained 5 times per week for 12 weeks and ingested their allotted test drink before and after training. Although no differences in strength were observed between groups at the end of the training period, there was evidence of a greater increase in muscle mass in the milk group than in either of the other two groups. Therefore, there is some proof that the repetition of a practice shown to achieve better acute synthesis of protein will result in long-term benefits. This is encouraging, but more studies are needed before firm recommendations for protein intake can be provided to athletes.

New Ideas on Fat Loss for Athletes

Many people consider obesity to be a community health problem that can be prevented or treated with exercise. In fact, even those who undertake many hours of exercise each day may still have a real or perceived need to reduce their body fat levels; it is often the primary reason for athletes to seek the services of a sports dietitian. Of course, only a small number of athletes need to lose body fat for health reasons. Some athletes have aesthetic motives for wanting to reduce body fat levels; these range from a personal desire to improve appearance in tight-fitting or skimpy Lycra uniforms (e.g. female athletes in team sports, swimmers, beach volleyball players) to actual performance enhancement in sports in which a subjective judgment of physique contributes to the final outcome (e.g. body building, gymnastics, diving, figure skating). In many sports, however, physical improvements in performance are associated with increasing the athlete's power to weight ratio (enhancing the ability to move body mass, particularly against gravity) or reducing the athlete's size (enabling complex movements to be completed in a small space). The first of these benefits is seen in sports such as distance running, cycling, high jumping and gymnastics, while the second is seen in sports such as diving and gymnastics. Finally, in other sports there are weight categories designed to create a 'level playing' field in which athletes of similar size, reach and strength compete against each other (e.g. combat sports, lightweight rowing, lifting sports). Most athletes do not arrive naturally at their optimum physique but must work to achieve it. This can become a particular issue following periods of weight gain, such as the off-season or while injured, when it is easy to develop an energy surplus.

Given the interest in fat loss as an issue in sports nutrition, it is surprising that few studies have investigated different strategies in athletes. Instead the major focus has been on practices for rapid reduction in body weight in weight division sports ('weight making') involving dehydration and fasting [16]. A reduction in body fat levels requires the achievement of an energy deficit, either by reducing energy intake, increasing energy expenditure or by combining both methods. The suitability of these various options will vary according to the athlete but may pose some problems: additional exercise may increase the risk of injury or otherwise interfere with the athlete's primary training, while restricting energy intake may reduce the athlete's ability to meet the nutritional goals for optimum training. Furthermore, the loss of body fat is usually accompanied by a loss of lean mass: this is not desirable to most athletes. In addition to choosing the right time within their periodized calendar to undertake loss of body fat, the athlete will want to choose a method that minimizes the negative impact on their training capacity or performance. The review by Phillips and Zemel [17] provides some potential strategies to achieve these goals.

In the general population, there is some evidence that hypoenergetic diets lower in carbohydrate and higher in protein may promote the loss of body fat and retention of lean mass more than weight loss diets of the opposite macronutrient ratio [18, 19]. Other potentially beneficial strategies include the emphasis on carbohydrate-rich foods of low glycemic index [18] and an increased intake of dairy foods [20]. The evidence for these strategies comes from observational studies, animal trials, and some clinical trials in overweight populations. Investigation in athletic populations seems warranted, although some modifications or periodization may be needed when these strategies are in opposition to the athlete's sports nutrition goals (e.g. carbohydrate needs for refueling or performance). The potential benefits of increased intake of dairy foods on fat loss via both calcium-dependent and calcium-independent mechanisms are of interest, however, since dairy protein may also assist with the athlete's goals for protein synthesis related to training adaptations. In fact, there is currently a high level of interest in dairy products in sports nutrition circles; products like flavored milk can provide useful quantities of fluid, electrolytes, protein and carbohydrate in a practical form for consumption in the athlete's diet [21].

Increasing Substrate Availability by Increasing Fat Utilization

Fat and carbohydrate have a reciprocal relationship as substrates for exercise. However, the total body stores of carbohydrate are limited, whereas even the leanest athlete has sufficient fat stores in the muscle and adipose tissue to support very lengthy exercise. A well-known adaptation to training is to increase the capacity for fat utilization at the same absolute and relative work rates compared with pretraining values. Since training alone does not equip the body to achieve maximum rates of fat utilization, it makes sense for athletes to consider other strategies that might further enhance fat use during exercise. Unfortunately, unlike animals such as rodents and migrating birds, fat oxidation cannot sustain the very high rates of power generation required for high-intensity exercise in humans. Instead, fat oxidation is inhibited at exercise intensities above ~75% of maximum aerobic capacity. Nevertheless, an increased use of fat to sustain low-moderate intensity exercise may spare glycogen as a substrate for the high-intensity work undertaken during an event or for prolonged events which are limited by glycogen depletion. Potential opportunities include strategies that acutely increase free fatty acid (FFA) concentrations during exercise, or more chronic strategies that re-tool the muscle to increase its capacity for fat oxidation (i.e. increases in fatty acid transport into the muscle, uptake into the mitochondria or capacity for β-oxidation).

Spriet [22] provides an elegant overview of the regulation of fat metabolism during exercise and recovery, identifying the potential points which could be targeted to allow an increase in fatty acid utilization during exercise. The first option of increasing the plasma concentrations of FFAs and their delivery to the muscle can be achieved by relatively short periods of fasting or restricted carbohydrate intake, as well as by acute or chronic consumption of a high-fat diet. High-fat diets can certainly improve exercise capacity in the rat [23, 24], but the early studies of Christensen and Hansen [25] showed a reduction in endurance in men fed a high-fat, low-carbohydrate diet for several days. In such studies, it is theoretically impossible to separate the effects of the high fat intake from the absence of carbohydrate consumption. Short-term fasting can isolate the effects of carbohydrate withdrawal; this strategy also increases endurance capacity in the rat [26], but generally results in a decreased exercise tolerance in man [27]. One explanation for the failure of these strategies to enhance exercise capacity in humans is that although fat oxidation is increased, at best this only compensates for the reduced contribution of carbohydrate rather than enhancing total substrate availability, and in most cases it is unable to meet the shortfall caused by reduced body carbohydrate stores. Fat oxidation also requires a higher rate of oxygen consumption for the same energy demand, so may not be appropriate when oxygen delivery is limited.

A high-fat meal just before exercise could theoretically increase blood FFA availability without sacrificing body carbohydrate stores, but the digestion and absorption of fat is slow. A more effective way to achieve this outcome involves infusion of a lipid source with heparin injections, but this is not practical for athletes to use in the field (and it contravenes the WADA regulations). The ingestion of medium-chain fatty acids during exercise offers another potential way to increase plasma FA since these fats are digested, absorbed and transported into the muscle cell and mitochondria more efficiently than their long-chain counterparts. However, the practicality of this strategy is also limited since the amounts that can apparently be tolerated during exercise without causing gastrointestinal distress are too small to cause any worthwhile sparing of muscle glycogen [28]. A final dietary strategy known to acutely increase plasma FFAs is the ingestion of caffeine. Although an increased fat utilization and concomitant glycogen sparing was one of the mechanisms first suggested to explain the beneficial effects of caffeine on exercise capacity, more recent studies have shown that this effect is short lived (disappearing by ~20 min into exercise) and not universally observed [29]. In summary, there does not appear to be a simple and practical way for athletes to achieve an acute manipulation of plasma FFA levels to benefit exercise performance.

Retooling the muscle to enhance FFA transport across the muscle or mitochondrial membranes or to upregulate β-oxidation pathways offers other options to usefully enhance fatty acid utilization during exercise. Carnitine supplementation has been promoted for many decades as a potential enhancer of fatty acid oxidation (and fat loss, by the weight loss industry) due to its role in transporting fatty acids into the mitochondria. This has occurred without any proof, until recently, that increased carnitine intake is taken up by the muscle. There is emerging evidence that intake of supplemental carnitine with insulin-stimulating carbohydrate-rich meals may slowly increase muscle carnitine concentrations [30]. The functional outcome of this finding requires further investigation, and the commercial possibilities will surely drive this forward.

Longer term exposure to a high-fat, low-carbohydrate diet has been shown to cause chronic adaptations in the muscle to increase its capacity for fat oxidation at rest and during exercise; these changes include increases in fatty acid transport proteins and enzymes involved in fat mobilization, uptake and oxidation [31]. A couple of studies have reported that 2–4 weeks of intake of such a diet by trained individuals was associated with enhanced capacity for endurance exercise, but the majority of studies have reported no benefits to exercise endurance or performance, and a longer term study (7 week) actually found a compromised adaptation to the training process [31]. Certainly, the ability to train at high intensities is impaired by a low-carbohydrate diet, and there may be some alteration of the adaptive response to the same training stimulus. For this and general health concerns, long-term exposure to a high-fat diet is not recommended to athletes. However, changes in the muscle in response to a high-fat diet and high-volume exercise appear to be achieved in about 5 days in well-trained subjects and are maintained in the face of restored carbohydrate availability, at least in the short-term [32]. Thus, the concept of dietary periodization has been proposed, involving rapid adaptation to a high-fat diet followed by carbohydrate loading and carbohydrate feeding during exercise; this offers the potential benefits of the combination of high carbohydrate availability with spared use. Again, despite clear evidence of altered substrate use during exercise, no benefits to exercise capacity or performance have been detected with this strategy [33]. One explanation for this apparently incongruous finding is that the exposure to a high-fat (low-carbohydrate) diet not only upregulates fat utilization during exercise, but downregulates glycogen use due to a reduction in activity of the pyruvate dehydrogenase complex [34]. The practical implication of this finding of *impaired* rather than *spared* glycogen use is a reduction in performance of high-intensity bouts within an exercise protocol [35]. This is likely to be of major practical importance in the world of sport in which the decisive moments in even ultra-endurance events lasting many hours involve high-intensity activities. In summary, there appears to be a sophisticated reciprocal relationship between fat and carbohydrate utilization during exercise that can be manipulated to show interesting outcomes in terms of exercise metabolism. However, the practical outcomes do not favor performance benefits and may even impair critical aspects of sports performance.

Adaptation of the Gut and Exogenous Fuel Supply

In exercise lasting longer than about 40–60 min, ingestion of carbohydrate can enhance performance [36]. Ingested carbohydrate must first be emptied from the stomach into the small intestine where it is absorbed and made available to the working muscles. The rate of intestinal absorption seems to be the main limitation to the provision of exogenous carbohydrate to the working muscle during exercise. High rates of oxidation of exogenous carbohydrate can be achieved whether this is ingested in liquid, semi-solid, or solid form [37, 38], though there may be performance advantages to liquid formulations which can simultaneously provide fluid as well as carbohydrate [39]. Ingestion of mixtures of different carbohydrates, including glucose and fructose, which are absorbed by different pathways, may allow maximization of intestinal absorption rates, and can lead to higher rates of exogenous carbohydrate oxidation during exercise: this has been shown to result in better endurance performance [40]. In events that last up to 2 h, a carbohydrate intake of up to about 60 g per hour might be recommended. When exercise lasts more than 2 h, slightly greater amounts of carbohydrate (up to 90 g/h) may be preferred. When such high rates of carbohydrate ingestion are attempted, they should consist of a mix of multiple transportable carbohydrates, such as glucose:fructose or maltodextrin:fructose.

The gut is capable of rapid adaptation to periods of feeding and fasting, and is highly responsive to changes in the composition of the diet. The maximum rates of carbohydrate absorption that can be achieved may be enhanced by a period of adaptation to a high-carbohydrate diet. In a study of highly-trained athletes, a group who consumed glucose during each of their workouts over a 4-week training block increased their ability to oxidize this carbohydrate, while muscle oxidation of carbohydrate consumed during exercise remained constant in a matched group who did the same training with ingestion of water [41]. The design of this study could not distinguish whether the adaptation was achieved by a higher intake of carbohydrate or the specific intake of the carbohydrate during exercise. However, it seems sensible to advise athletes who plan to consume carbohydrate during competition to practice this in training to train their behaviors and race plan, as well as to take advantage of this gut adaptation.

Recovery and Replenishment of Fuel Stores: Training Harder versus Training Smarter

The adaptations to a training program are proportional to the training load, so nutrition strategies that allow greater intensity of training and allow faster recovery between training sessions are important to maximize the benefits. For many years, athletes have been encouraged to consume a high-carbohydrate diet during periods of intensive training and to begin the process of carbohydrate ingestion soon after the end of a training session [12]. These strategies are designed to allow the athlete to train hard and, indeed, some training studies have shown that such strategies achieve a better performance outcome at the end of a block of intensive training or help to reduce the effects of a block of overtraining [33].

Recent investigations of the muscle metabolic response to a training stimulus have found, in fact, that compared with a comparable situation featuring high muscle glycogen content, an acute bout of (endurance) exercise commenced with low muscle glycogen stores results in a greater transcriptional activation of enzymes involved in carbohydrate metabolism (i.e. the AMP-activated protein kinase, GLUT-4, hexokinase and the pyruvate dehydrogenase complex), and an increase in adaptive responses favoring fat metabolism [42, 43]. In other words, training with low carbohydrate availability might enhance the response to the same exercise stimulus – or 'train smart'. This has led to another concept of dietary periodization where an athlete would 'train low' to promote a greater training response, before switching to high carbohydrate availability for competition when optimum performance was required [42]. The watershed study undertaken by Hansen et al. [44] intrigued sports scientists and coaches/athletes alike by purportedly providing evidence to support this view. Previously sedentary men consumed a carbohydrate-rich diet while training one leg with a 'two a day' protocol (two sessions every second day, with a rest day between) and the other leg with single daily training schedule. Although each leg completed the same training load and increased its maximum power output equally, the 'two a day' leg which commenced 50% of its training sessions with a low glycogen concentration, showed a greater enhancement of its capacity to work at ~90% of pre-training maximum power output. While these findings have significant scientific merit and possible application for exercise programs targeting metabolic improvements and health outcomes, there is potential for misunderstanding by athletes and coaches.

First, it should be noted that train low does not require a long-term adherence to a low-carbohydrate diet, and there are a number of options for reducing carbohydrate availability in the training environment that might enhance adaptation to the training stimulus. These include exercising after an overnight fast, consuming only water during prolonged training sessions, withholding carbohydrate in the hours after exercise or restricting carbohydrate below the fuel requirements of the training load [45]. Such protocols differ in the duration of the period in which the body is exposed to a low carbohydrate environment as well as the focus on reducing endogenous and/or exogenous muscle fuel sources. As described above, the two a day training protocol of current interest involves a carbohydrate-rich diet, and uses the rescheduling of training sessions to achieve a low glycogen environment for some of the sessions, but possible supercompensation of glycogen during the rest day [44].

Second, the transference of changes in enzyme or protein content of the muscle cell to athletic performance needs to be questioned. To date, the train low literature has found that undertaking some exercise sessions with low glycogen concentrations or low exogenous carbohydrate availability can enhance the metabolic adaptations associated with training, even in well-trained individuals, but fails to provide a performance enhancement over a conventional training diet with high carbohydrate availability [46]. The final issue of importance is the consideration that train low strategies may cause some negative outcomes. A common finding from several train low studies is that capacity for training or training intensity may be impaired in sessions undertaken with low carbohydrate availability [47, 48]. This is important; coaches typically prescribe training sessions in which athletes are required to work at intensities/speeds/power outputs that are higher than their 'race pace'. Intuitively, a sacrifice of the capacity to train at high intensities should be made with reluctance until there is evidence that this does not impair performance. Finally, the effect of repeated training with low carbohydrate status on the risk of illness injury and overtraining needs to be considered [45].

Of course, most elite athletes practice an intricate periodization of both diet and exercise loads within their training program, which may change within a macrocycle or microcycle. Either by intent or for practicality, some training sessions are undertaken with low carbohydrate status (overnight fasting, high-volume training involving several sessions in the day, little carbohydrate intake during the workout), while others are undertaken using strategies that promote carbohydrate status (more recovery time, post-meal, carbohydrate intake during the session) [45]. Therefore, in real life, elite athletes already undertake a proportion of their training with low glycogen content. It makes sense that sessions undertaken at lower intensity or at the beginning of a training cycle are most suited to, or perhaps, least disadvantaged by train low strategies. Conversely, 'quality' sessions done at higher intensities or in the transition to peaking for competition are likely to be best undertaken with better fuel support. Athletes may, by accident or design, develop a mix-and-match of nutrition strategies that achieves their overall nutrition goals, suits their lifestyle and resources, and maximizes their training and competition performances.

Hydration and Salt Balance

Major disturbances of cell volume have profound effects on cellular metabolism [49]. Cell swelling will favor anabolic reactions, including protein synthesis and glycogen synthesis, while cell shrinkage will encourage these reactions to proceed in the opposite direction [50]. It is also apparent that metabolic activity within the cell or in other tissues can alter the distribution of water between the intracellular and extracellular space. During intense exercise, the concentration of the products of glycolysis will rise sharply: changes in glycogen concentration will have little effect on the osmolality of the intracellular space, but the concentration of phosphorylated intermediates and of pyruvate and lactate can rise markedly. Muscle lactate concentration can exceed 25–30 mmol/kg after intense exercise [51], and the rise in intracellular osmolality will cause the rapid movement of water into the active muscles leading to cell swelling and the initiation of compensatory mechanisms.

There is clearly potential for the athlete to exploit these mechanisms to promote desirable metabolic outcomes and to minimize unwanted effects. At present, however, our understanding does not allow practical recommendations to be made.

Conclusions

Current areas of discovery in sports nutrition include the interaction of nutrition and exercise on muscle protein synthesis, the nutritional environment for optimum training adaptations, the gut limits on providing exercising muscle with a supply of exogenous carbohydrate, and the manipulation of cell metabolism by changes in cell volume. We presently know that the ingestion of small amounts of protein after an exercise bout will promote net muscle protein synthesis to enhance the adaptive response to the session. This response can be maximized by ingestion of about 20–25 g of high-quality protein that provides about 10 g of essential amino acids. Endurance training on a carbohydrate-restricted diet will enhance the capacity for fat oxidation and may enhance the adaptive processes taking place in muscle. However, the downside includes a reduced capacity for training at high intensities as well as impairment of pathways promoting carbohydrate utilization. In well-trained athletes, at least, there is no evidence of performance improvements from strategies to 'fat adapt' or train low exclusively. However, there may be opportunities to include individual training sessions or blocks of training within the athlete's periodized training program to integrate the benefits of training with reduced carbohydrate availability. Intestinal absorptive capacity may limit the supply of exogenous carbohydrate during exercise, but this can be trained by following a high-carbohydrate diet and perhaps also by ingestion of carbohydrate during training. Such adaptations will allow the athlete to have better opportunity to supply additional sources of carbohydrate to enhance performance during events lasting more than 2–3 h. Manipulation of hydration status has profound effects on cellular metabolism, but the available evidence does not yet allow identification of effective strategies that can be applied by the athlete. Over the coming years, we expect to see refinements of this knowledge to allow athletes to fully exploit it to achieve their sporting goals.

References

1 Maughan RJ: The relationship between muscle strength and muscle cross-sectional area and the implications for training. Sports Med 1984;1:263–269.
2 Hopkins WG, Hawley JA, Burke LM: Design and analysis of research on sport performance enhancement. Med Sci Sports Exerc 1999;31:472–485.
3 Burd NA, Tang JE, Moore DR, Phillips SM: Exercise training and protein metabolism: influences of contraction, protein intake and sex-based differences. J Appl Physiol 2009; 106:1692–1701.
4 Tipton KD, Gurkin BE, Matin S, Wolfe RR: Non-essential amino acids are not necessary to stimulate net muscle protein in healthy individuals. J Nutr Biochem 1999;10:89–95.

5   Kimball SR, Jefferson LS: Signaling path-
    ways and molecular mechanisms through
    which branched-chain amino acids mediate
    translational control of protein synthesis.
    J Nutr 2006;136(suppl 1):227S–231S.
6   Moore DR, Robinson MJ, Fry JL, et al:
    Ingested protein dose response of muscle and
    albumin protein synthesis after resistance
    exercise in young men. Am J Clin Nutr 2009;
    89:161–168.
7   West DWD, Burd NA, Coffey VG, et al:
    Rapid aminoacidemia enhances myofibrillar
    protein synthesis and anabolic intramuscular
    signaling responses after resistance exercise.
    Am J Clin Nutr, in press.
8   Wilkinson SB, Tarnopolsky MA, MacDonald
    MJ, et al: Consumption of fluid skim milk
    promotes greater muscle protein accretion
    following resistance exercise than an isoni-
    trogenous and isoenergetic soy protein bev-
    erage. Am J Clin Nutr 2007;85:1031–1040.
9   van Loon LJC, Gibala, MJ: Dietary protein
    to support muscle hypertrophy; in Maughan
    R, Burke L (eds): Sports Nutrition: More
    Than Just Calories – Triggers for Adaptation.
    Nestlé Nutr Inst Workshop Ser. Nestec,
    Vevey/Karger, Basel, vol 69, 2011, pp 79–95.
10 Bodybuilding.com. 5 ways to get lean with
    protein. http://www.bodybuilding.com/fun/
    planet38.htm; accessed on 23 Nov 2010.
11 Atherton PJ, Etheridge T, Watt PW, et al:
    Muscle full effect after oral protein: time
    dependent concordance and discordance
    between human muscle protein synthesis
    and mTORC1 signaling. Am J Clin Nutr
    2010;92:1080–1088.
12 Coyle EF: Timing and method of increased
    carbohydrate intake to cope with heavy
    training, competition and recovery. J Sports
    Sci 1992;9:29–52.
13 Borsheim E, Cree MG, Tipton KD, et al:
    Effect of carbohydrate intake on net muscle
    protein synthesis during recovery from
    resistance exercise. J Appl Physiol 2004;96:
    674–678.
14 Koopman R, Beelen M, Stellingwerff T, et al:
    Co-ingestion of carbohydrate with protein
    does not further augment post-exercise
    muscle protein synthesis. Am J Physiol
    Endocrinol Metab 2007;293:E833–E842.
15 Hartman JW, Tang JE, Wilkinson SB, et al:
    Consumption of fat-free fluid milk after
    resistance exercise promotes greater lean
    mass accretion than does consumption
    of soy or carbohydrate in young, novice,
    male weightlifters. Am J Clin Nutr 2007;86:
    373–381.
16 Burke LM: Practical Sports Nutrition.
    Champaign, Human Kinetics, 2007.
17 Phillips SM, Zemel MB: Effect of protein,
    dairy components and energy balance in
    optimizing body composition; in Maughan
    R, Burke L (eds): Sports Nutrition: More
    Than Just Calories – Triggers for Adaptation.
    Nestlé Nutr Inst Workshop Ser. Nestec,
    Vevey/Karger, Basel, vol 69, 2011, pp 97–113.
18 Abete I, Astrup A, Martinez JA, et al: Obesity
    and the metabolic syndrome: role of dif-
    ferent dietary macronutrient distribution
    patterns and specific nutritional components
    on weight loss and maintenance. Nutr Rev
    2010;68:214–231.
19 Krieger JW, Sitren HS, Daniels MJ,
    Langkamp-Henken B: Effects of variation
    in protein and carbohydrate intake on body
    mass and composition during energy restric-
    tion: a meta-regression. Am J Clin Nutr
    2006;83:260–274.
20 Zemel MB, Shi H, Greer B, et al: Regulation
    of adiposity by dietary calcium. FASEB J
    2000;14:1132–1138.
21 Roy BD: Milk: the new sports drink? A
    review. J Int Soc Sport Nutr 2008;5:15.
22 Spriet LL: Metabolic regulation of fat use
    during exercise and in recovery. In Maughan
    R, Burke L (eds): Sports Nutrition: More
    Than Just Calories – Triggers for Adaptation.
    Nestlé Nutr Inst Workshop Ser. Nestec,
    Vevey/Basel, Karger, vol 69, 2011, pp 39–58.
23 Miller WC, Bryce GR, Conlee RK:
    Adaptations to a high-fat diet that increase
    endurance in male rats. J Appl Physiol
    1984;56:78–83.
24 Simi B, Sempore B, Mayet M-H, Favier RJ:
    Additive effects of training and high-fat
    diet on energy metabolism during exercise.
    J Appl Physiol 1991;71:197–203.
25 Christensen EH, Hansen O: Zur Methodik
    der respiratorischen Quotient-Bestimungen
    in Ruhe und bei Arbeit. Skand Arch Physiol
    1939;81:137–179.

26 Dohm GL, Tapscott EB, Barakat HA, Kasperek GJ: Influence of fasting on glycogen depletion in rats during exercise. J Appl Physiol 1983;55:830–833.

27 Maughan RJ, Fallah J, Coyle EF: The effects of fasting on metabolism and performance. Br J Sports Med 2010;44:490–494.

28 Jeukendrup AE, Saris WHM, Brouns FR, et al: Effects of carbohydrate (CHO) and fat supplementation on CHO metabolism during prolonged exercise. Metabolism 1996; 45:915–921.

29 Chesley A, Howlett RA, Heigenhauser GJF: Regulation of muscle glycogenolytic flux during intense aerobic exercise following caffeine ingestion. Am J Physiol 1998;275: R596–R603.

30 Wall BT, Stephens FB, Constantin-Teodosiu D, et al: Chronic oral ingestion of L-carnitine and carbohydrate increases muscle carnitine content and alters muscle fuel metabolism during exercise in humans. J Physiol 2011; 589:963–973.

31 Hawley JA: Fat-adaptation science: low-carbohydrate, high-fat diets to alter fuel utilization and promote training adaptation; in Maughan R, Burke L (eds): Sports Nutrition: More Than Just Calories – Triggers for Adaptation. Nestlé Nutr Inst Workshop Ser. Nestec, Vevey/Karger, Basel, vol 69, 2011, pp 59–77.

32 Burke LM, Hawley JA, Angus DJ, et al: Adaptations to short-term high-fat diet persist during exercise despite high carbohydrate availability. Med Sci Sports Exerc 2002; 34:83–91.

33 Burke LM, Kiens B, Ivy JL: Carbohydrates and fat for training and recovery. J Sports Sci 2004;22:15–30.

34 Stellingwerff T, Spriet LL, Watt MJ, et al: Decreased PDH activation and glycogenolysis during exercise following fat adaptation with carbohydrate restoration. Am J Physiol Endocrinol Metab 2006;290:E380–388.

35 Havemann L, West S, Goedecke JH, et al: Fat adaptation followed by carbohydrate-loading compromises high-intensity sprint performance. J Appl Physiol 2006;100:194–202.

36 Jeukendrup AE: Nutrition for endurance sports. J Sports Sci, in press.

37 Pfeiffer B, Stellingwerff T, Zaltas E, Jeukendrup AE: Carbohydrate oxidation from a semi-solid carbohydrate gel compared to a drink during exercise. Med Sci Sports Exerc 2010;42:2038–2045.

38 Pfeiffer B, Stellingwerff T, Zaltas E, Jeukendrup AE: Oxidation of solid versus liquid carbohydrate sources during exercise. Med Sci Sports Exerc 2010;42:2030–2037.

39 Below PR, Mora-Rodriguez R, Gonzalez-Alonso J, Coyle EF: Fluid and carbohydrate ingestion independently improve performance during 1 h of intense exercise. Med Sci Sports Exerc 1995;27:200–210.

40 Currell K, Jeukendrup AE: Superior endurance performance with ingestion of multiple transportable carbohydrates. Med Sci Sports Exerc 2008;40:275–281.

41 Cox GR, Clark SA, Cox AJ, et al: Daily training with high carbohydrate availability increases exogenous carbohydrate oxidation during endurance cycling. J Appl Physiol 2010;109:126–134.

42 Baar K, McGee SL: Optimizing training adaptations by manipulating glycogen. Eur J Sport Sci 2008;8:97–106.

43 Hawley JA, Burke LM: Carbohydrate availability and training adaptation: effects on cell metabolism and exercise capacity. Exerc Sport Sci Rev 2010;38:152–160.

44 Hansen AK, Fischer CP, Plomgaard P, et al: Skeletal muscle adaptation: training twice every second day vs. training once daily. J Appl Physiol 2005;98:93–99.

45 Burke LM: Fueling strategies to optimize performance: training high or training low? Scand J Med Sci Sports 2010;20(suppl 2): 11–21.

46 Philp A, Burke LM, Baar K: Altering endogenous carbohydrate availability to support training adaptations; in Maughan R, Burke L (eds): Sports Nutrition: More Than Just Calories – Triggers for Adaptation. Nestlé Nutr Inst Workshop Ser. Nestec, Vevey/Karger, Basel, vol 69, 2011, pp 19–37.

47 Yeo WK, Paton CD, Garnham AP, et al: Skeletal muscle adaptation and performance responses to once a day versus twice every second day endurance training regimens. J Appl Physiol 2008;105:462–470.

48 Hulston CJ, Venables MC, Mann CH, et al: Training with low muscle glycogen enhances fat metabolism in well-trained cyclists. Med Sci Sports Exerc 2010;42:2046–2055.

49 Lang F: Effect of cell hydration on metabolism; in Maughan R, Burke L (eds): Sports Nutrition: More Than Just Calories – Triggers for Adaptation. Nestlé Nutr Inst Workshop Ser. Nestec, Vevey/Karger, Basel, vol 69, 2011, pp 115–130.

50 Lang F, Busch GL, Ritter M, et al: Functional significance of cell volume regulatory mechanisms. Physiol Rev 1998;78:247–306.

51 Sahlin K, Harris RH, Nylind B, Hultman E: Lactate content and pH in muscle samples obtained after dynamic exercise. Pflugers Arch 1976;367:143–149.

52 Davies J, Dickerson J: Nutrient Content of Food Portions. Cambridge, The Royal Society of Chemistry, 1991.

53 Holland B, Welch AA, Unwin ID, et al: McCance and Widdowson's the Composition of Foods, ed 5. Cambridge, Royal Society of Chemistry, 1991.

54 Paul AA, Southgate DT, Russel J: First Supplement to McCance and Widdowson's the Composition of Foods. London, Her Majesty's Stationery Office, 1987.

Subject Index

fuel utilization during exercise
    effects 60, 61
intake recommendations by duration
    of endurance events 5, 6, 9, 10
loading 2
protein coingestion effects 83, 84
types 3–6
Carnitine palmitoyl transferase-1 (CPT-1)
    exercise response 23, 35
    fat metabolism 43
    high-fat/low carbohydrate diet
        response 64, 76
CD36
    exercise response 57, 58
    low glycogen training response in
        muscle 21, 23
Cell volume
    athletic performance
        considerations 124, 145
    cytosolic osmolarity balance 116–118
    exercise effects in muscle 129
    gene expression response 120,
        121
    insulin effects 127, 128
    metabolism
        cell volume influences on
            metabolism 119, 120
        metabolism influences on cell
            volume 123, 124
    regulatory cell volume
        decrease 119
        increase 118, 119
        isovolumetric regulation 127
    signaling 121–123
Citrate synthase, low glycogen training
    response in muscle 21
Cyclic AMP response element-binding
    protein (CREB), exercise response 22

Dairy foods
    anti-obesity effects
        branched-chain amino acids 103
        calcitriol 102, 103
        calcium 102, 110
        clinical studies 103–105
    food types and effects 113
    milk protein 111, 112

Dehydration, see Cell volume

Energy-restricted diet
    composition 100
    fat loss strategies for athletes
        138–140
    weight loss and body composition 99,
        100

Fat, see also Obesity; Triglyceride,
    intramuscular
    free fatty acids
        availability enhancement 46
        chain length effects on
            metabolism 48, 49
        exercise effects 55
        metabolism 42, 43
    high-fat/low carbohydrate diet
        adaptation
            muscle adaptation
                enhancement 66–69
            training interaction in training
                adaptation 65, 66
        carbohydrate restoration effects on
            fuel utilization during
            exercise 61–65
        fat oxidation enhancement
            mechanisms 64, 65
        fuel utilization during exercise
            effects 60, 61
    loss strategies for athletes 138–140
    metabolism
        recovery 49, 50
        regulation overview 40–44
    oxidation
        enhancement in well-trained
            athletes 46–49
        training effects during exercise 44,
            45
    substrate use by exercise intensity 39,
        40
    utilization enhancement 140–142
Fatty acid translocase, see CD36
Free fatty acid, see Fat

Glycerophosphorylcholine (GPC), cell
    volume regulation 118

Glycogen
  carbohydrate intake effects on
    synthesis 17
  glycogenolysis 20
  training with low glycogen
    athlete viewpoint 25–28
    molecular viewpoint 20–25
    prospects for study 28, 29

High-fat diet, *see* Fat
Hormone-sensitive lipase (HSL), exercise
  response 23, 34, 35, 42
Hydration, *see* Cell volume
3-Hydroxyacyl-CoA dehydrogenase, low
  glycogen training response in
  muscle 21

IDEAL study 108, 110
Insulin
  cell volume effects 127, 128
  exercise response 13
Intramuscular triglyceride, *see*
  Triglyceride, intramuscular

Lactate, consumption 15, 16
Leucine
  anti-obesity mechanisms 103, 105
  effects on energy partitioning between
    fat and muscle 99
  food portion sizes and
    composition 136, 137
  insulin response of proteins 112
  muscle protein synthesis effects 91, 101

Milk, *see* Dairy foods
Mitogen-activated protein kinase
  (MAPK), cell volume response 120,
  122
Muscle, *see* Adaptation; Protein;
  Triglyceride, intramuscular
Myocyte-enhancing factor-2 (MEF2),
  exercise response 24
Myoinositol, cell volume regulation 118,
  120

Nuclear respiratory factor-1 (NRF1),
  exercise response 24

Obesity
  dairy food anti-obesity
    mechanisms 102–105
  fat loss strategies for athletes
    138–140

Peroxisome proliferator-activated
  receptor-γ coactivator-1α (PGC1α)
  dietary fat availability and muscle
    adaptation enhancement 67, 86
  low glycogen training response in
    muscle 21–23, 25, 33, 35, 36
  training response 45, 56
Peroxisome proliferator-activated
  receptors (PPARs)
  dietary fat availability and muscle
    adaptation enhancement 67, 69
  low glycogen training response in
    muscle 21, 24, 25, 32, 33
Phosphoinositols, cell volume
  regulation 123
Potassium channels, cell volume
  regulation 119
Protein
  dietary
    acute versus long-term anabolic
      response 85–87, 92, 93, 101
    carbohydrate coingestion
      effects 83, 84
    energy-restricted diets 100,
      101
    food portion sizes and amino acid
      composition 136, 137
    intake recommendations 82, 135–
      138
    milk protein 111, 112
    role before, during, and after
      training 135–138
    sources 82, 83, 93
    timing of ingestion 84, 85
  muscle synthesis and breakdown after
    exercise 80, 81, 89–91, 94
Pyruvate dehydrogenase (PDH), high-fat/
  low carbohydrate diet response 64,
  73

Regulatory cell volume, *see* Cell volume